I'm not in control:
Coping with Alzheimer's disease

I'm not in control: Coping with Alzheimer's disease

Nancy Swiston

iUniverse, Inc.

New York Lincoln Shanghai

I'm not in control: Coping with Alzheimer's disease

iUniverse books may be ordered through booksellers or by contacting:

iUniverse
2021 Pine Lake Road, Suite 100
Lincoln, NE 68512
www.iuniverse.com
1-800-Authors (1-800-288-4677)

Because of the dynamic nature of the Internet, any Web addresses or links contained in this book may have changed since publication and may no longer be valid.

The views expressed in this work are solely those of the author and do not necessarily reflect the views of the publisher, and the publisher hereby disclaims any responsibility for them.

ISBN: 978-0-595-45013-8 (pbk)
ISBN: 978-0-595-89328-7 (ebk)

Printed in the United States of America

I need to thank everyone who helped me with my mom. Without each and every one of them, we never could have done all that we did. I will be forever indebted to them all, but this book is dedicated to one very special lady. This is dedicated to my Aunt Anna. She was one of the most inspirational women I knew, with the exception of my mother. We were a constant "three-some". She adored my mother and loved her as a true sister (when in fact she was my father's sister). She helped me and was always there for me to guide, comfort, inspire and make me be the best I could be. She made me look at myself and question my own feelings. She was there every step of the way with my mom's illness. She was my sounding board for many hours of conversations, tears, and many more tears. She was the only person who knew everything from day one because she was always with us. It was because of her continual urging that I started to write down my thoughts and experiences. I wish I could take credit for the whole idea—but I'm sure that it was all hers. I can't tell you how broken hearted I was to lose her a year before my mom. If I could make a wish for all caregivers it would be that you could have an Aunt Anna in your life. She was that someone special in your family that knows you better than you know yourself. This is done in memory of Anna Chapo—with all my heartfelt thanks to her.

Section 1—Before

Why this book?

It isn't until something changes that we appreciate what we have. I am a worrier by nature but never in a million years would I have thought my world could be turned upside down so completely. My life had been good and I definitely wasn't prepared for what was going to happen. Things aren't going to change and of course a parent will never change. My mom was so sharp; she was a retired insurance rater. Numbers were nothing for her. She did our income tax every year. It wasn't until much later that I saw signs of her just getting forgetful. It was even more later on that she began doing odd things at odd times—just not her.

My mom is a totally amazing woman. She is very independent and very self-sufficient. I had been out on my own for about 7 years (what stuff I had accumulated in that short time). So after I return home with all of my possessions, the house is truly overflowing. The house is crowded but we are together. At that point she doesn't need me to live with her; it is just more economical for both of us. I live with my mom and I work full time in a business office at a school. It is a job that I enjoy doing. My mom and I are good friends, who tend to disagree (probably because we are both strong willed and stubborn) and our disagreements include just about everything. With that being said, please know that I love her dearly. And so the story begins …

Why am I writing this article? I need to write down my thoughts to help myself cope and because I want to help others who are in a similar situation. If you are reading this article, your life isn't easy and I know it. There are no answers. Just possibly some guides to coping with the situation. Your life will be changing constantly and be assured that it won't be getting better. There is no better, the best you can hope for is to just hold your own. Your loved one will be changing and you need to be in the changing mode yourself. I feel one of the most important things to remember is that although your loved one is changing, maybe even daily; you need to **love the person they are now—right now**. You can remember how they were—but take a realistic look at the person they are currently. It's definitely no one's fault. It's not their fault nor is it your fault.

Alzheimer's disease—this illness is robbing you of the loved one you have only in memories now. They are not the same person they were, but they need your love now more than ever before. Your strength and your determination are vital to their well-being. Someone once told me, that there is a book in all of us, and that is where it usually should stay. Going against their better judgment, I am writing this article anyway. My reason for doing this, is in hopes of helping someone deal with his or her life a little better. If it helps you at all, even in some small way, then my goal is reached.

Why the title "I'm not in control" you may be asking yourself? When you are growing up, you strive to be in control of your life. I was definitely a control freak and felt that I controlled my own destiny. We think we know what we want and we can make things happen. We all can't wait to be grown up. Life is full of possibilities. There are so many decisions, college choices, career choices, job opportunities and so forth—we pick the path we want to follow. We are in control, or so we think. At least that is what I thought, and boy was I wrong!

Author's note: Please forgive me for using different tenses throughout this book, probably over half this book and all of the journal was written while my mother was alive. About a year after she passed away, I was drawn again to this book. I added some parts and edited others, so the tenses tend to be both present and past throughout this book. I apologize for any confusion I may have caused.

The initial realization

You start to see strange things happening. I had noticed she wasn't changing her clothes. I was doing the wash and I thought she was just trying to lessen the amount of clothing to be washed. I tended to believe that, like so often, she was thinking of the work and me. This wasn't the case.

I was leaving her lunch on a plate in the refrigerator. All she had to do was take it out and eat it. I would get home, and what I found was unbelievable. I had cut the sandwich in quarters and she would eat the top of one section, a couple bites out of another section and pulled the cheese off a totally different section. Normally, someone would just eat a quarter or two if they weren't hungry. This was not normal behavior.

I went to the post office to mail some bills that my mom had done and I realized that the slips that tell where they go, weren't placed right, so no address showed in the window. I took them to work with me. There I opened them and put the pages in correctly and then mailed them. I'm thinking she must have been in a hurry. This wasn't the case.

Often I would call her from work and she wouldn't pick up the phone. I would worry and call my best friend. My friend would run over there to check on her. Mom would be there and just not realize she needed to pick up the phone. There were many more incidents like the ones I have mentioned and I knew she had to be supervised. You won't notice these little things at first, but after you finally realize, you will be able to look back and see all the signs very clearly.

The cost of daycare was enormous, so I had my aunt spend a day or so each week with her at our home. My aunt loved being with her. She said that she was amazed that mom would constantly ask for me at 4 o'clock every day. "Where's Nancy? Shouldn't she be home now?" My aunt knew that mom couldn't tell time, yet every day at exactly the same time it would start and mom would get agitated. This is nothing mysterious; this restless period is known as "sundowners". Another problem was that my mom refused to take off her socks; I couldn't get her to remove them. She even kept them on at night. Trust me when I say there was no touching those socks. Thanks to the urging of my aunt we were able to finally get those off. Her feet were horrible and my aunt and I soaked them. I never saw feet so bad. Getting my mom to do anything she didn't want to do was nearly impossible. There were many arguments and many disagreements. The beginning stages of dementia are difficult because they have more good moments than the bad ones. They think they know best. I also believe that being a daughter makes it tougher—kids are supposed to listen to parents and not the other way around. My aunt's support was a Godsend in so many ways.

The health system trap

When my mom got sick that first time and wound up in the hospital, the realization and the gravity of the situation followed quickly. The hospital said the family needed to stay with her night and day because of the dementia. Being the sole caregiver (and her only child!), I stayed both day and night. I saw a sharp decline in her condition. After the slight heart attack, she formed blood clots. They had her on blood thinners. While she was in the intensive care unit, they took a blood sample from the groin area and they never applied pressure, so she had a huge hematoma. The whole experience was a true nightmare. They insisted that I had to apply to Medicaid. So instead of being with my mom at the hospital, I am running all over the place. At home I found mom's metal box, the one with the important papers. She was so organized; all the envelopes were marked, if only there had been papers inside. Who knows where she had put the papers. So I'm running around trying to get copies of birth certificates, marriage licenses, my dad's death certificate and so forth. What a huge waste of time, when I needed to be with her constantly. She was so scared. She was constantly screaming my name, calling out for me. She needed to learn to walk again. They told me she couldn't do rehab in the hospital because, due to the dementia, she wouldn't follow directions well enough and for long enough. Now looking back I'm not sure that was the case, I maybe should have pushed harder.

Rule one: Please remember, don't second-guess your own feelings—you know your loved one the best. She did follow direction then, but needed constant repetition. I believe she could have done the rehab in the hospital with that constant repetition and I now wish I had made a bigger issue of it. It is so hard, because you want to be "nice", so they will be "nice" to your loved one.

Rule two: Beware of the hospital's social worker. I learned that the hard way. The social workers at the hospital, work for that hospital, and that is their first concern. You can listen to them and consider what they are telling you, but the bottom line is that they work for the hospital and have the hospital's best interest at heart—not yours. Never forget that important fact. They know the exact number of days that are allowed to the patient (through their insurance) and can use that information to their advantage. What the social worker is telling you will be biased, so take it for what it is worth.

Rule three: Most importantly, do your own research and investigating, don't rely on anyone to give you your options. You need to know what your options are.

Rule four: Always have a game plan. I called all the nursing homes that did rehab and were decent and then did visits to them to see their facilities. After my initiating the process, they did their evaluations on my mom. They all said that she wasn't capable enough. The nursing homes are leery of accepting a patient for short-term rehab because they could be forced to keep the patient after the rehab is over.

In my mom's case, the hospital placed her in a section of the hospital that I refer to as limbo land for many weeks. I call the ward where she was kept "limbo-land" because everyone in that wing was waiting for nursing home placement. Mom was just sitting there in the hall, lined up with all the others. It was a horrible situation, everyone just there, with their minutes of physical therapy each day that really didn't do any good. The hardest thing was to see my mom in a "posey". It is a restraining cloth garment that keeps their arms tucked along side their bodies. She was constantly struggling with the posey and it was horrible to watch. My cousin said she was like Houdini, as she would somehow manage to escape the cloth restrain. My mom's strength was unbelievable. It was so sad to see her tied up and I can't help but wonder if better training for dealing with dementia patients wouldn't show better results. The hospital was in charge. Her struggling was cruel, and that extreme frustration for her couldn't have done any good.

I was told they were sending my mom to a nursing home for short-term rehab. I visited the nursing home to which they were sending my mom. I cried. It wasn't a good place. It didn't matter; they sent her there anyway. I refused to go and sign the hospital's release papers; it didn't matter, and then they sent her there anyway. This really illustrates that total loss of control. I was told that her days covered by her insurance and Medicare had run out and the hospital had to release her because it was costing money. Believe me, they know exactly how many days are covered and they kept her exactly to that last day. What a health system we have—they are milking the system for all that it is worth. My heart goes out to all the poor people that are caught up in the health system trap. The caregivers have to be aware so they can play the game. Moral of the story: who was in control? You can bet it wasn't me. It didn't matter what I wanted or what I did—I was so NOT in control.

Looking back only one good thing happened from that whole ordeal. When the hospital discharged my mom, no actual bill was incurred. So the nursing home said that I had to reapply for Medicaid and I refused. That was the all-important loophole that I needed to get my mom out of that horrible place. Luckily for me, I used that trump card. They insisted that I apply to Medicaid and I insisted that I wouldn't, the battle began. They said that mom belonged in the nursing home permanently. My plan was to bring her home. When her rehab days were up I wasn't backing down. They said that I would never be able to work full time myself and take care of mom at home. They actually came to the house to see if she would be in a safe environment. If it proved to be unsafe, they could have refused to release her. I was ready, bring them on and let them scrutinize me. Just give me a challenge—I'll jump right on it and I did. Remember I did say that I had inherited my mom's stubbornness and strong will. Thank God, I was able to get us out of the system. I was going to show them! In my heart, I felt that I fought the system and won. I do realize that the system may vary from place to place, but that is why it is so important to find out what you are up against in your area. Find out how things work where you live because only then will you be able to make correct decisions for you and your loved one.

Well, I was happy with my small victory. I had mom home with me. I'm not going to lie and say it was easy, because that would be far from the truth. My mom had declined greatly and she was very hard to handle at first. It truly took weeks to get mom calmed down at home. She was almost like a wild animal—I used lots of hugging and soothing words. She was physically in good shape but mentally she was worse than ever. Nights were nearly impossible. I bought room-darkening shades to totally keep the daylight out. When I put her down she was agitated and she wanted to get back up. I would try to talk her to sleep, trying to relax her. Keeping her in the bed was a great challenge. My friend gave me a side support railing-thing that you put on a toddler's bed. I used that and it worked for a short time. Until mom realized that she could simply push it out and get up. I ended up putting dining room chairs up against the side bed railing and laid cushions on them for me to rest there while she would fall asleep. In the nursing home she was getting up in the middle of the night and falling, her knees were in horrible shape, all bruised and bloody. My mission was to heal up those knees. I'll say it again, it wasn't easy, and the nights were extremely endless. But those knees were looking much better in a short time.

Her mental condition had declined so much at the nursing home. I feel it was because the nursing home had removed her Aricept, so she hadn't received any for all those months. When I had questioned the doctor at the nursing home, I was told that my mother didn't suffer from Alzheimer's disease; therefore she didn't need that medication. Funny that after bringing her home, giving her the drugs prescribed by our family doctor, like the Aricept—there was improvement. Imagine that. I find this very interesting and it really makes you wonder how long she would have lasted had she remained in that nursing home.

The stages

You, the caregiver, will be going through an evolution. You will find yourself beginning to question everything. You will be going through many different stages. First there is disbelief, then despair, and then anger. This first level is dis-belief. It just doesn't seem real and maybe things won't be as bad as they say. Then the full impact of everything hits you. I was angry and that anger wasn't good. I was angry because my mom was sick, she would never be the same again. I was angry because this whole situation was going to change my life completely. Why her? Why me? Why us? I had to let go of the anger. On many occasions, my aunt told me to let the anger go so it wouldn't eat me up inside. That is much easier said than done. My mother's friend next door is the exact same age as my mom, so why didn't it happen to her? I needed to accept that certain things were simply out of my control. Here was that control thing again! Accepting that fact has helped me deal with the whole situation a lot better. It is a very sad but true fact. The anger and the acceptance of the situation have to occur for you to be able to move on in any way, shape or form. You have to deal with it first, so you can deal with it for them. You need to gather your wits about you because you are in the fight of your life, for their life.

Section 2—During

To tell or not to tell

I was told that as soon as you know your loved one has Alzheimer's, you should tell all your friends, family and neighbors. That way they can help you if your loved one would "wander". With others knowing they can help you watch your loved one. In my way of thinking, there was another way to look at all this. I personally chose to tell very few. My mom was a proud, independent person and I felt it gave her more dignity for a longer period if I told only a couple people who needed to know. At this point, dignity was one of the only things I could give her and I wanted her to have that. I did what I felt was right at the time. Looking back I see that it could have been a mistake. With the disease the person may be saying things that are unfavorable of you to others—who would expect this to happen, not me. My mom adored me—I knew that. However, my mom had this horrible disease, she wasn't herself. Surprisingly, my mom told horrible things to my aunt who was afraid to tell me because she knew they were untrue, and I would only get upset. My Aunt Anna meant well. So my aunt never told me any of the things that my mom had said to her. This wasn't good in the long run. You have to remember that neighbors and or family get a distorted view. For example, my mom would scream bloody murder every time that I wanted her to get into the shower (she didn't like water running over her head), so needless to say, every time was a very, very "loud" incident. Looking back, it probably sounded like I was killing her. My solution was to stop the sound. This was easy. I actually got air conditioning for the house, so I wouldn't have to open any windows. I assume that my mom had talked to some of the neighbors. I had a neighbor that thought I was a despicable person and even told me so on different occasions.

In my case a cousin-in-law wrote a letter to Senior Protective Services to get protection for my mother. The investigators came to the house to question my mom and right away they realized the situation. All it did was badly upset my already confused parent. Now she was sure that this person who notified the authorities "hated" her. I was sure that they hated me—so here we were arguing over whom they hated more. What a waste of time and energy that was. All of a sudden she was on medication for an upset stomach, something that she never needed before her visit from the investigators. Thanks to that "relative", and I use that term loosely, all my mother got was more confused and even more agitated. There had to be a better way for someone who was truly concerned to handle it. I feel that my cousin should have contacted a mutual family member to intervene before contacting the authorities. Please remember if you think something is not right, be very careful before contacting someone who could make things even worse. Try talking to the person involved. If my cousin had approached me, I would have explained the situation. My cousin was in such a state of mind that she thought that my mother could do some babysitting for her niece. So she was the one who wasn't seeing the real situation. This whole thing was so ridiculous. Even if I had told her, she wouldn't have probably believed me because you "see what you want to see"—but it would have been nice if she had given me the opportunity to explain. The true ironic part is that my cousin still believes that she knows better. According to her, the intervention made me change my ways and thanks to her, she saved the day. This was definitely not the case. Supposedly the investigators were to report back to her and tell her things were fine—unfortunately my cousin knew better than them all. How do you deal with this?

You need to expect the unexpected. You truly are not going to know what your loved one is going to do. I want to share another story; I had put in for a vacation at work and was looking forward to the time off. We have family in Syracuse and they were anticipating our visit. Well, the morning we were supposed to leave, my mom decides for absolutely no reason that she isn't going to go. So I insisted she was. Now remember when I said that no one tells my mom what to do, well I wasn't kidding. Mom got upset, called the police and then she threw the phone at me. She normally wasn't a violent person; she was just very upset with me. The police came and so did those neighbors that know what a horrible person I am. It was a very uncomfortable situation. I didn't tell anyone about mom's condition that day—to tell that nosey neighbor would have been like telling the world. We didn't get to Syracuse that day or the rest of my time off. Later, my cousin John in Syracuse passed away and that would have been the last time I would have seen him alive. The decisions you make will be tough and so are the consequences. These stories illustrate that things will happen to put you in a bad light and you have to be able to deal with these situations accordingly.

I can say that I don't care what people think of me, but I do care. It's hard to swallow, when you know bad things are being said about you. I made difficult decisions and I did my best. Be prepared that no matter what you choose to do, as the caregiver—people may not see how things really are anyway or even believe what you are telling them. You have to learn to take it in stride. Some people are bound to think the worst. You know how you are doing—you have to not care what anyone else thinks. Again, this is much easier said than done. Just remember that it doesn't matter what anyone else thinks, you have to do as you see fit and you are the one who has to live with yourself. I have heard that it can be good to be an only child. By being an only child, all of the decisions are made by me alone. With several siblings, agreeing on different matters could have been difficult. The sibling living in town versus the sibling out of town could see things very differently. Again with many siblings, the major responsibility may all fall on only one anyway. These decisions are hard; but remember they not only involve you but also your loved one.

My lesson learned from all this: Be prepared for trouble either way. If you tell people, they probably won't believe you. In the beginning stages, your loved one can seem very normal and rational at times. They will probably think you are making it up and just want your parent put away. I saw some signs at the start, and I was told that I was overreacting. My mother mistook someone for someone else. I was concerned. I was told that they looked alike. My mother got confused about where she lived (half her life she lived right across the street). She wanted to go home across the street. I was concerned. I was told after all she did live there a long time, she was just confused. As I said before, it's so important to go with your instincts. You know your loved one the best. If you feel there IS a problem—there probably is one, and there has been one for quite a while. Remember, we tend to not see a situation clearly when we are so directly involved in it. We as caregivers also only see what we want to see. A very dear friend told me that she saw signs of dementia with my mother and didn't tell me because she knew I wouldn't believe her (her husband also had dementia at the same time). People that are involved with people, who have dementia, probably can see signs much sooner than the average person. I wish she would have told me but I'm afraid that she is correct in saying that I wouldn't have seen it and quite possibly would have resented her for saying it. It is a very "touchy" situation and you are walking on a very fine line.

People didn't notice and I didn't say. My mom was so normal. She had an endearing habit of calling everyone "honey". Before the illness, she really did know everyone's name. However, due to this habit, remembering names wasn't noticed—everyone was honey. I'll never forget one day my aunt, my mom and myself stopped at McDonald's for lunch. We got coffee, and we all ordered hamburgers. I saw mom struggle with money in paying. I felt she should live as normal as possible, so I carried two purses, so she would have hers. It was so hard to see her struggle with these mundane tasks. Anyway, it was so funny when we sat down to eat my mom asked why there were two small packages of honey on her tray (like the jelly that comes in those little packs). So the three of us are trying to figure it out and all of a sudden it hits us. She must have called the guy honey, twice and he thought she was asking for some. It was something that we often laughed about afterwards.

See the doctor quickly

My advice is to get your loved one to a doctor as soon as possible. There are special doctors that specifically deal with dementia in older people. If you don't want to go to a specialist, just get them to their family doctor. Remember that time matters, so don't delay. They can test to see if there is a problem. Our family doctor tested my mom right in his office. There was a series of questions and it was truly amazing to watch. She sat there, and you could see her thinking so hard to come up with the answers. The simple math problems and clock diagrams had her completely baffled. I will never forget that day, when the doctor told her that she had Alzheimer's disease; there was absolutely no response from my mom. This statement is mind boggling, and there was no reaction. If I had any doubts in my mind about my mom's condition—they were gone at that moment. **The diagnosis of Alzheimer's disease is truly a death sentence**. It is fatal. I was heartsick, and my mom was totally unaware of what he had said, or the impact that statement would have on her life.

There are drugs that can make a difference. My mother was put on Aricept and also something for the depression. I got my mom to the doctor, possibly not as soon as I should have because I listened to others. Please learn from my mistakes. Do what your heart tells you—you know your loved one the best. Get them to the doctor to be diagnosed. When my mother was put on medication, there was an unbelievable change, she was "normal" again, and so I continued to say nothing to family and friends for the time being. Two of my mom's friends always picked her up on the last week of the month for the Senior Citizen Dinner Meeting. I didn't say anything to them for many months and it was a long time before they realized. My mom continued to go to the meetings with them for close to a year. When they finally asked me one day if there was something wrong with my mom, I did tell them. That was the end of the dinners for my mom. They no longer picked her up to go to the meetings anymore. So I'm glad that I didn't say anything sooner. I wanted her to have the most normal life possible for the longest possible time. Normal is familiar and familiar is good. I would do everything exactly the same again in a heartbeat.

Being their advocate

The definition of advocate is one called to the aid of another; one who pleads the cause of another. There are many difficult decisions to make and you are now the advocate for your loved one. With Alzheimer's your loved one can't tell you what is happening to them. I felt I had to be there as much as possible, to really know what was going on. It seemed that overnight the role of the parent and the young child had been reversed. Now it was my turn to watch out for my mother. You can't take this role of advocate lightly. You are their spokesperson, their mouthpiece—THEIR EVERYTHING.

They no longer know what is best for them. I found myself "child proofing" the house. I made towels for her to wear at mealtime, because she was eating the paper napkins. I sewed Velcro on the hand towel to attach it behind her neck—they worked great. They no longer know what is food and what isn't. No small objects sitting on the table anymore because everything goes into her mouth. When she would eat a paper napkin, it was impossible to get it out; she would refuse to open her mouth. I don't use Styrofoam cups for the same reason. My mom's first day care place would give them drinks in Styrofoam cups. Why would a place dealing with folks that have dementia—use those cups? I could never understand that. I was called at work one day because my mom had taken a bite out of her coffee cup and wouldn't open her mouth so they could get it out. I am not trained in any form of health care, but I truly was amazed that these folks couldn't see that their cups were the problem in this case and not my mom.

At home I was making improvements to the house all the time—I tried to do a project a year. These improvements were so costly. I wanted all floors to be level, no little step-downs. No area rugs to trip on. I installed wall-to-wall carpeting throughout the house. I put in a separate walk-in shower in the bathroom. I'm pretty sure that I'm the only house on the block with two showers in the same bathroom. However, to step into a tub was impossible for her to do anymore, hence the walk-in shower did the trick. Steps to get into the house were also a hurtle. I had to put a wooden ramp out the back door. The building of the ramp was a costly but necessary project. I moved the washer and dryer to the main floor of the house, so I could watch her at all times. No chance of her falling down the cellar steps while I'm throwing in a load of wash. So the washer and dryer were put in a closet on the main floor. I was having trouble with the ramp on the wheelchair van laying flat. When it flipped out of the van it was getting caught up on our brick driveway, so I had a concrete driveway poured (done in sections, because of the cost). My dad had laid the brick driveway and it was so hard for me to see that go. You do what you have to do. I had a chain link fence put up to help keep mom in the yard. The list goes on and on. Every year a new project, always something else to do. You need to make whatever changes you can to make your situation better. In helping them you are also helping yourself to help them.

I have already said that your loved one will be constantly changing; we need to change ourselves and often even the things around us will also need to change. That ramp that I put at the back door did undergo many changes over time. Originally, I had an open step in one section of the ramp/deck. Mom had trouble with her knees. At first, mom could do a step, going down backwards using her footed cane. I wanted the step there so she would be able to use it. We would practice the step. The old saying of "use it or lose it" is so true. At the end it was taking three of us to get her down the step. However, it got to be too hard to do after a while. Then one day mom went towards the step with the walker, I called the contractor and had him temporarily put a board up until a gate could be put on the top of the step. Next thing, when mom was in the wheelchair (she would walk the chair around with her feet) and she would go all around the deck—it was good exercise, so I encouraged it. One day she turned and started going down the ramp section of the deck. I called the contractor again. This time he put a bar that could be flipped down—to stop access to the ramp section. When mom could no longer hold her feet up, I had to put the foot holders on the wheelchair. Then I had trouble making the turns in the ramp section. So again the contractor was called. This story of our ramp, illustrates exactly how your needs will change over time. What is fine at one time will need revisions again and again as time goes by. If nothing else I have learned to roll with the punches, take things in stride and just make it work.

Be your own inventor

God works in strange ways and I truly believe that I was suppose to go to a classroom and listen to a guest speaker one day while I was at work. The teacher had invited me to sit in her class. Wilson Greatbatch had invented the pacemaker and my mom had a pacemaker. I wanted to meet him and hear this man speak. He had pacemakers with him and he passed them around the classroom. I held a pacemaker in my hands and was amazed. I see the slight bulge in my mom's chest and now I had learned what this was and how it worked. However, the pacemaker lessons weren't going to be the big lessons that I was to walk away with on that fateful day. This man was brilliant, he was an inventor, and he said that anyone could be an inventor. He was trying to motivate these young children. He was speaking to a class of 4th and 5th graders at the school—but I felt his words were meant for only me. Anyone could be an inventor—I could be an inventor. The day I spent in Mrs. Raven's class and listening to this man has changed my outlook and my life. His logic will be engrained in me forever. Our overall outlook can determine our whole viewpoint in life.

You need to become your own inventor. You need to look at any situation throughout your day, and try to figure out a way to make it easier. I feel this philosophy is the best advice I have ever been given in my entire life. I try to look and see what I can do to make my life (taking care of my mother) easier for me. The key is to look at a small section of your day and analyze it. With small being the key word in that statement. Analyze that small task. Small tasks can be made easier and you will be surprised how much smoother your day can go. Dealing with a small task also helps in diminishing that totally overwhelming sensation of the whole situation. In the mornings I have to have my routine down to a science—every single second counts. I need to do things the same way and in the same order each day. This routine is as important to my mom as it is to me. It makes things familiar to her, and helps me not to forget to do something in my haste. Thanks to that day in that classroom, I did become an inventor and that skill helped me more than I can say. You can be an inventor, too.

Dealing with work

Getting to work on time is one of my biggest challenges, so therefore I'm under great pressure to accomplish this task. It's so hard to stay optimistic when dealing with an employer. My mother is the number one thing in my life, with work running a close second. I need to take care of my mom and I needed my job to help me financially to do just that. Work doesn't understand; they want you at your desk at a certain time no matter what it takes. Dropping my 150-pound mother off at daycare isn't as easy as taking a small child that you can just pick up and carry in if they are giving you a hard time. My baby is very big and still has a mind of her own at times. I do the best I can in the mornings.

I was always very nervous and upset mornings. I found myself sweating profusely as I struggled with her in the mornings. My best friend came over every morning for years to help me with mom. I had tried to get an aide and it was impossible. They would only come for a minimum of 2 hours and I had to be out of the house before 7 am. Getting help isn't easy; no aide was going to come here at 5 am. My friend was wonderful and came over every morning to help me; I was blessed to have her help. When I say every morning, I truly mean that, weekdays, weekends, every day. She was the sister I never had and the other daughter that my mom never gave birth to. Calling her my best friend just doesn't do it justice. She would help us, only to hurry home to get her own son ready for school. She couldn't understand why I was so frustrated mornings, but she had no clue of all the grief I would get at work. I would be climbing on the bed and I usually ended up changing my clothes before I could leave for work. Stress does wreak havoc on your body. Lately I have come to the conclusion that you can only do your best—so why get more upset on top of it. I have my morning schedule and I follow it the best I can. Moral of this story is—remember just do your best, make it easier and keep it routine!

Work is such a difficult situation to explain. I really believe that we need to educate people in general about the illness of Alzheimer's disease. I think people think of it in a very light sense. It's just something that happens to older people. It's normal, it's just aging. It's like forgetting where you put your keys, or forgetting someone's name or just being slightly confused. It encompasses so very much more. It's about forgetting who everyone is and about forgetting who you even are. It's about forgetting how to do simple tasks, like standing, walking and even how to go to the bathroom. It's about forgetting how to comprehend directions. It's about forgetting how to hold a spoon or even how to swallow. It's about eating Styrofoam cups and paper napkins, not knowing what is food and what isn't. It's about forgetting everything! It's about this slow deadly process that is killing you. It is fatal! Telling others that my mom has Alzheimer's disease—they can't begin to imagine the vastness of all this. I was continually getting into trouble at work for being late. I had been up and constantly running around for about 5 hours before I even got to my desk in the morning. The reality was, that I was simply happy to eventually make it there, period, and to finally be able to sit down. We were so very "not on the same page", and it was a huge problem. Don't expect anyone to really understand what you are going through—they never will.

I think the biggest problem is that Alzheimer's disease is such a long-range illness. It's not like having an operation where you are out, then recovering and then returning. There is no quick time table and no way of predicting when things were going to happen. At one point, my supervisors were having me meet **weekly** with them to discuss my situation. It was so humiliating! I will never forget those horrible meetings. No one will ever know how that made me feel. A fortuneteller I'm not—who knows what lies ahead. My dealing with my mom's illness was a constant and ongoing issue, and now work was putting the pressure on. Answers—who had answers—certainly not me? I was trying to cope as best as possible; it was so frustrating and I was trying to explore every avenue. Purchasing that costly "used" wheelchair van had been a necessary item and not a frivolous purchase. I was struggling to get mom out of the car at daycare and was consequently late. There were many days of being late and being so frustrated. With the used van, things were much easier. I was trying my best. At one of the weekly meetings, I had suggested using an hour or two of my vacation days each day, so the workday could be shorter and I could get to daycare sooner (daycare was requesting it). The answer I got to my request was, if I didn't need to work 8 hours a day, then maybe my job shouldn't be full-time. They just wouldn't bend an inch.

I feel I need to mention, that one day I found an article on my desk titled "how to choose a nursing home". I couldn't believe my eyes. What a way to start my day. How could anyone do that? Those decisions are very hard and very personal. I tried to not take it personally and tried to put a positive spin on it. In their defense, I believe that they were trying to help. However, they weren't helping; I wanted my mom at home with me. No one knows what's best for me. I can't emphasize enough, don't expect anyone to really understand what you are going through.

Not only will work not understand but you will also see this in friends, family and others. On a whole I noticed that my friends were better about the dealing with it. My mom's friends were scared, they were the same age, and they couldn't handle it. Be prepared because all people will act differently now. A boyfriend that I had gone out with, on and off for about 13 years, asked me to marry him (but he implied that we needed to put my mom in a nursing home). Make me make a choice—no choice there. I picked my mom. How he could expect me to put her in a nursing home was unbelievable. At the same time he was struggling with a difficult teenager and he wanted his daughter at home with him. Wouldn't you think he would have sympathy for my passion to keep my mom home with me? He didn't, not at all! He walked away and never looked back. The funny irony on this was that when my mom was well, she adored him. Towards the end of our relationship, he wouldn't even come over to my house until after I had put her to bed. There were many nights when we were watching a movie on TV that I would fall asleep and he would make snide remarks. Part of me loved him and part of me was relieved when he made no more demands on my time. My mother always said, "All things happen for a reason". I believe that our relationship wasn't meant to be. I think everyone can be a friend when times are good; it's the bad times that show you your true friends. That saying of every daughter wants to find a man like her father is true; well this guy just couldn't come close. Please remember to not let others influence what you want to do. The struggles were constant whether at home or at work. One thing was certain; I never doubted my commitment to my mom for a second.

Not everyone at work was judging me. A nurse that worked in my building gave me a half sheet of paper one day. She said that she was thinking of me. I read the paper, took it home and hung it on the wall in my bedroom. It was called "The 10 Absolutes of Caregiving for Alzheimer's Patients". It follows ...

Never **argue**, instead, **agree**.

Never **reason**, instead, **divert**.

Never **shame**, instead, **distract**.

Never **lecture**, instead, **reassure**.

Never say, **"remember"**, instead, **reminisce**.

Never say, **"I told you"**, instead **repeat**.

Never say, **"you can't"**, instead say, **"do what you can"**.

Never **command** or **demand**, instead **ask** or **model**.

Never **condescend**, instead, **encourage** and **praise**.

Never **force**, instead, **reinforce**.

(Notes from a communications seminar by Jo Huey, Greater New Orleans Patient and Family Service Committee, as reprinted in the Alzheimer's Association of Western NY Newsletter, Vol. 3, 1998) These are very powerful words and something that needs to be referenced often. It is still hanging on my bedroom wall.

A dear friend of mine gave me a book to read and it truly helped my work situation in a way nothing else could do. Her daughter had recommended it to her and she passed it on to me. I highly recommend everyone reads "Suzanne's Diary for Nicholas" written by James Patterson (Warner Books Edition, copyright 2001, pages 23-24). It is a wonderful love story. But the most important fact was that there was a story within a story. I found the telling of the five balls to be a remarkable thought to hold on to. I quote "Imagine life is a game in which you are juggling five balls. The balls are called work, family, health, friends, and integrity. And you're keeping all of them in the air." To me this book really illustrated our busy lives and the juggling of these different areas. He told the reader that the work ball was rubber; however, all the other ones are made of glass. If the glass balls are dropped they will be damaged or even totally shattered. These glass balls are precious and need to be handled very carefully. The work ball is rubber and that ball will bounce if dropped. This story of the five balls put everything into the proper perspective. This balance of the balls, this balance of your life is the most important concept. This wonderful idea has kept me going and kept me in the right frame of mind. Many times at work I found myself talking to myself saying "rubber ball, rubber ball". This unusual story made all the difference to me. Please don't forget, if it gets dropped that work ball will bounce. I found that getting that balance of life is the true key of dealing with work.

Find a confidant

Do find someone to confide in. You need to find your own support system. Call your branch of the Alzheimer's Association to see what is offered in your area. These people are experts. They have probably heard it all before and they want to help you. You need to let them. They are only a phone call away to answer every question. Use all the resources you can to the fullest. Go to any seminars that you hear of—even if you only pick up a small pointer or two, it could make a big difference in your life. Find out where there are support groups and see if they can help you. Go to a support group and see how it feels, I had to go to a couple before I found a group with which I was comfortable. Sometimes they offer care for your loved one, while you attend. Try many. Try everything. What helps one person may not help another. Find out what works best for you. But do get a support structure in place upon which you can rely as soon as possible.

You need to talk to someone to release your feelings. The important thing to consider here is that only a person in a similar situation is going to really understand. Be prepared—most friends and relatives will back away. This shying-away is hard to deal with from supposedly people that care. My hardest thing was not to take that to heart. I find this is one of the most difficult things to accept. People are afraid. People don't know what to say or do. It's not that they don't care; they just don't want to be near it. My mother was loved and admired by all she touched. She was so giving, so caring and so loving of others. She was everyone's "favorite" aunt. She was the one who remembered all birthdays and anniversaries with a card and a kind word. She told the most wonderful family stories and in a way that no one else could do. Listening to her, you felt like you were standing right there next to her. These stories could keep people entertained and laughing for hours at a time. Most of my mother's closest friends never stop to see her anymore. I'm sure it was hard for them to deal with. If you are the same age or older, you have to be thinking that this could happen to me. But isn't it hard for any of us to see someone we love in such a different state. I certainly don't like seeing how my mom is now. But she is how she is, and it is so important that we accept and make the best of it. One of my mom's friends was here on many occasions and you will find that certain people will still try to make an effort. My nature was to not ask for any help from anyone. It's important to realize that you need to accept any help offered. Don't be a martyr.

At this point I want to mention an angel who came into our lives. My mom's best friend lived right next door for my entire life. About 3 years ago she moved and sold her house. The young woman who moved in—I really believe that she was an angel sent to us. At first, she would come over and help me shovel the ramp and or driveway to get mom into the house. But it wasn't the physical things; it was the emotional things that were the true blessing. She was drawn to my mom. She truly adored my mother. She never knew my mom as she used to be, only the later person with dementia. She formed such an attachment with my mom, that it was simply astounding. You could truly see that my mom adored her also. This relationship shows that in spite of the dementia, personality does come through. She certainly didn't need us to keep her busy, she was married with a husband and three children. But this amazing woman, found time to come over every evening to help me walk my mom. This story does emphasize that fact I had said—it is so important to love the person they have become. They are not the person they were, but they are something to treasure all the same. Love the person they are now. This relationship will never cease to amaze me. As I have said everyone adored my mom, but this woman never knew the way she was. That strong personality still came out, even with the dementia. She would bring her daughter over and my mom always loved children and you could see my mom's eyes light up. My new neighbors truly were a blessing to us.

Search for help

Help will come from a variety of places. My biggest source of help was from the Alzheimer's Association. As I have said, they are the experts. They have many programs in place that can be a huge comfort. I called often and was helped greatly by Jennifer Baran, a worker at my local chapter. She was wonderful. She made sure that others read my letters. She actually knew my mom from her day-care. She sat with my mom the day that I spoke at the Town Meeting. She went above and beyond her responsibilities for us. The Alzheimer's Association is a great resource. The workers there know what you are going through. The Call Center will take calls 24/7, 365 days per year. The Call Center has 30,000 inquiries per month. They can help in 140 different languages. It's someone to talk to at any hour of the day or night and the local chapter does follow up calls the next day. Problems will occur at all hours and the need to talk to someone will be there. The Safe Return Program is another blessing. Currently more than 148,000 people are registered with this program. Your loved one can be registered, and you will have peace of mind that if they wander, a system is in place to help find them. About 60% of people with Alzheimer's disease will wander. The

Alzheimer's Association trains and works hand in hand with the local police departments. It is a known fact that if a person has wandered off and isn't found within 24 hours, they could undergo great harm or even die. It is a very effective program and it has a 98% return rate. Both of these programs are so important in providing safety to the demented person and peace of mind to the caregiver.

Although I called the chapter often, I didn't register my mom with the Safe Return Program, only because she couldn't wander. Due to her knee injuries, she reached a point where she needed assistance standing. Later I learned that I should have registered her anyway, because the caregiver also wears a bracelet and this tells that someone is depending on you. It is a very important service and one you should utilize.

There was only one time that I lost my mom. It's ironic that the only time I couldn't find my mom was when she was in the horrible nursing home for rehab. One day I went there directly from work and couldn't find her in her room. I asked the nurses on the floor and they said that she was probably one floor down in the activity room. I went there, and she wasn't there. I looked and looked. I finally went down the hallway, and I saw an empty wheelchair by the public restroom. I knocked on the door and I heard mom's voice. I opened the door, and there she sat on the toilet. She had been trying to stand up and couldn't. I'm guessing that she had been there a VERY long time because her clothes were drenched with sweat. No one noticed that mom was missing, and no one noticed the empty wheelchair in the hall. I couldn't get her out of there quick enough. What a place!

Our County Senior Services have also been a source of information. The person, who is assigned to my mom, has been very helpful to me. Mom's caseworker had a person from Jewish Family Services come to my house to counsel me. This was really good, because going somewhere can be difficult, so that person comes here to my house and when it's convenient for me. She recently had come after I had called a hospital supply store to get a Hoyer Lift to help me get mom up from bed in the mornings. I had a rented one and had it in my living room. She mentioned that she had seen one that day in the Buffalo News. I went online and saw the ad. I called this person the next day from work; he lived two minutes from where I work. He had lost his wife the week before. I was able to buy his lift for what it would have cost to rent the other one for just a couple months through mom's health insurance and Medicare (big co-pay). This counselor was a great help with many different items. She encouraged me to write letters. She was a great source of information. Remember to use all resources that are available to you.

The Red Cross or your local Lions Club chapters could have loan closets where you can borrow equipment that is needed. I was lucky enough to get a hospital bed from the Lions Club when it started to get difficult to get mom out of the bed. You don't need to buy everything, see if things can't be borrowed. I was told that the Red Cross gives classes that would also help us in general with aspects of caregiving. Find out what is in your neighborhood.

Computers are a source of so much information. I know I spent many hours on line exploring one subject or another. I went to libraries and read books. If you don't own a computer, the libraries have ones that can be used. The only stupid question is the one that isn't asked. Don't stop looking for answers.

Keep your life going in various directions

As a caregiver, it's important to keep your life going in a couple other directions while you are going through the care-giving ordeal. I unfortunately still needed to work full time (approximately 14 years to go until retirement). As much as work can be a hassle most times, it also can be a haven. It's the needed break in the routine of caregiving that you so desperately need. The people I work with are my friends, family, and confidants all in one. Working revives me to deal with things better when I pick her up at the end of the day. I have become a much more organized person, I had my "to do lists" at work and then I come home and have my lists to do here also. It's ironic, although I was very tied up with my caregiving tasks, I found I got a lot more accomplished then. That saying, "if you need something done, ask a busy person"—is definitely true. I was busier than I'd ever been and yet I was accomplishing so much more than I ever thought possible. My energy level surprised me, but at the end of the day I was totally exhausted.

Don't make the caregiving duty the soul purpose of your life because when something happens to your loved one, it will be impossible to deal with it. It's a good time to try to do something nice for someone else. Try to focus on other issues. Doing good deeds for others is good therapy for you. I find I want to help people. But most importantly I want to help people that are in a similar situation. There aren't many more things I can change in my life, but possibly someone can learn from what I've gone through. Thus, with the creation of this article, I'm writing down my thoughts and viewpoints hoping to help others. I know that every situation is going to be different but there will be some common parallels and I think it is always so important to be prepared. I have made many mistakes along the way—please learn from my blunders.

Don't forget to give yourself some "my time". You will be so much more content, if you take the time to do something that you enjoy. The happier you are, the better you will be able to be the needed caregiver that you are. You need to make time for yourself. I find my quiet times are after I have put her down at night and before I get her up in the morning. I try to do something I enjoy at those times. Make yourself read a book, take that bubble bath, do a game on the computer or whatever you feel like doing. You need to unwind; the caregiving task is very overwhelming. Make a point to talk to your confidant on a regular basis. It's important to know you're not alone. I'm very fortunate to have two people I talk to. All three of our situations are very different, but they are equally not good. At least we can understand and quite often give each other pointers and tips.

Living with your loved one is no easier or harder than the constant running to a nursing home. This I learned when my mom was in that facility for rehab for a few months. It was a horrible ordeal. Luckily my mom had a roommate that was fantastic. She was my eyes and ears for me when I had to go to work. She was 90 years old, but her mind was in excellent shape. The only problem is that when she told me something, I had to be very careful, how to deal with the situation without getting her into trouble for telling me. Your concerns and worries will be with you whether your loved one is at home with you or in a health care facility. Those concerns and worries don't stop and are ever present in either situation. Having your loved one in a facility can be even more stressful, just because you aren't there 24/7. I do feel truly blessed because I can still have my mom home with me. Having her here at her home is so very important to me. I truly believe that there is a future in providing services to people in there own familiar home situations. I would think that the government would provide help in the home versus the high cost of a nursing home. Doesn't it seem logical? How much money have I saved the government over the years? If I had applied to Medicaid when she was in for rehab, what would have over 5 years of nursing home care have cost? I find this financial aspect is very interesting. It's like we are punishing the caregiver who is trying to keep their loved one at home. The costs are huge—there are no tax breaks. Where is the incentive? Where is there any help?

If you have a friend and or family member who has dementia, please remember to stop and visit them, even if you can't really talk to the person anymore; your presence can mean so much. Those treasured visits can be a lifeline to that person. The socialization is vital. My mom was always better when there were people around. My mom always loved to be around people—to talk, laugh and tell stories. I feel that "company" is so very important. She loved people and she needs to still be around people.

There are Adult daycares out there

Adult daycare can be an answer. This was the answer for us, and that is one of the main reasons why I take my mom to a daycare. Even if I didn't work, I still feel that going to daycare is so necessary—the social interaction is crucial. Some people criticized me for dragging my mother out in all kinds of weather. But the important thing to remember is that they need to keep moving, getting up and going (especially to a person who has worked their whole life) it's a very natural thing to do. Try to get them involved in a daycare BEFORE they need to go. That way they will be familiar with the whole day care situation. It can be good for anyone to go to—even if only occasionally at first. They usually have field trips for the better health participants. Even going just a day or two at the beginning can make a big difference in the progression of the disease. I can't stress enough that the social interaction is so vital. I believe that without daycare in my mom's life, she would be much worse right now. It helps the communication skills. I also can't stress enough, by going to the daycare early on, they will be familiar with the surroundings and later they will be more at ease there. Familiar surroundings are very important and lessen the confusion later on. The cost can be a factor, see if the County is affiliated with any of the day care in your area. Possibly there are programs that are County funded that can help reduce the cost of this expense. Leave no stone unturned.

Get involved with the daycare. Stop in at different times to see what they are doing. Possibly you will need to try a couple different daycares till you find the one that is right for your loved one. Some daycares provide services like showers or bringing in hairdressers. Having a stranger do the shower thing can be a good thing. Often my mom was much better for others. I remember struggling in the kitchen trying to put curlers in my mom's hair or the struggles in the bathroom trying to get her in the shower at home. Letting others do these things can relieve much of your aggravation. Daycare can be a blessing for so many reasons. Take advantage of any services that are offered at the daycare.

Look for signs from your loved one. Remember they may not be able to tell you exactly how they are being treated there. Again, you are their advocate. Here are some questions to ask yourself: How are they acting when you drop them off? Are they hesitating getting out of the car because they don't want to go in? What is their reaction to the workers in the daycare? Are they smiling at the worker (or showing some other form of affection)? How is your loved one when you pick them up? Is your loved one anxious or nervous? This could be a result of the way they were treated throughout the day. My mom was VERY agitated and nervous when I picked her up, to the point where she wanted to open the car door as I was driving her home. I responded by buying a four-door car (with childproof locks on the back doors). However, when we changed daycares—my problem stopped instantly. My mom was thrown out of her first day care (the Styrofoam cup place) and it was such a blessing in the long run. She spent over 4 years at the next day care and she was very happy there. That first place had kicked her out because she wasn't good enough for a social daycare—then why did she last over 4 years at the next one? I can't help but wonder. The daycare set up is so important. The first place was a large room with many tables. In the second place it was designed so well, with many smaller rooms that gave it a "cozy" feeling. The office was set between the rooms with glass panels looking out on to both rooms. It was amazing to see that small rooms could have such an open feeling. These cozy rooms coupled with the same Corelle dishes that we use at our house; I'm sure made my mom feel right at home there. The wonderful staff was also a plus. The daycare change was good. All things probably do happen for a reason.

Remember you are now their eyes, look for signs. You need to know that they are happy and healthy when they aren't in your care. Do look for the signs; you will be surprised how much you can really learn from them. They don't need to talk to get a message across. You need to be observant on a very big scale. Another tip: use a different type of diaper on them than you bring to daycare (for changing), that way you can see if they have changed her without asking. During the week, the people at the daycare are with my mom more waking hours than I am. Weekends are my 24-hour periods. And I am emphasizing the 24-hour part of that statement. I sometimes gratefully look for Monday mornings to arrive because weekends do take their toll. That doesn't mean that I don't love my mother with all my heart, but the weekends are a long period to be on constant watch. At first the weekends really exhausted me, but I have found that all things get easier with time. Day after day, that constant repetition helps. You have to give situations and routines the time needed to adapt them to your life. It is so important not to give up, over time things do tend to get much easier, you just have to hang in there—as frustrating as it can be.

Going to daycare was an eye opener in many ways. With me being a "younger" caregiver, my heart goes out to a spouse caring for a spouse. I truly can't imagine physically doing what I am doing 20 years down the road. The physical wear and tear on a caregiver has to be so much harder when you are older. A child caring for a parent at least has age on their side. I remember driving up to mom's daycare and watching this little old man taking the wheelchair out of the back of his station wagon. Then he would lift his wife out of the front seat and place her in the wheelchair. My heart was so touched by his devotion. As I sat behind him in my used wheelchair van, waiting for my turn to pull up to the door, and with also being half his age, I actually felt guilty for having the van. Caregivers deserve a break and these items are so important to our task.

Tricks of the trade

To reiterate some points—it's important to combine the thoughts that I have already mentioned. Do things exactly the same from day to day. It helps both you and your loved one. The routine helps you not forget to do something and the person with dementia is more at ease with the familiar routine. Always try to think of a better way of accomplishing a task. It is important to always analyze a situation and come up with a way to make it simpler or quicker for you. One of my problems is always time in the morning. I was the sole caregiver, and I had a full time job. Every second counted in achieving my goal of getting to work on time. Little tricks like lining the garbage container in my mom's room with many grocery plastic bags inside one another. So when a wet diaper is placed in it, it can be closed up and taken out of the room right away. It was my version of the infants "diaper gadgets" that wrap up the used diapers. My goal was always to get my mother cleaned up and not have any odors in her room. The supermarkets have sprays that remove odors from the air and sprays that remove odors out of fabrics—take advantage of all the products out there. I have a shelf in my mom's room that looks like a shelf in the supermarket, full of many products that I stock up on when they are on sale.

Your local hospital supply store can be a wealth of information. There are many helpful gadgets like a handle for the bed (it goes between the mattress and box springs) to aid in getting up from the bed. They have a no-rinse body wash and no-rinse shampoos that will make the daily washing experience go much smoother. I adored the no-rinse body wash; it was so much better than using bar soap, no soap scum in the washbasin. Visit the store often; think of it as a resource of information. Ask to look at catalogs or brochures. Never stop trying to analyze a situation to find an easier way to do a task.

I wanted my mom to feed herself as long as possible. There are so many little things that can make the feeding process go more smoothly. I purchased very cheap placemats, which were made of the material that people use to stop things from moving. This grip-y material holds the plate in place much better. I also found larger plates that had a lip, so you could use the side of the plate to push the food on the spoon or fork. I also purchased a small child's fork and spoon set. It had a thick foam handle, which was easier to handle. So my mom has her

Scooby Do silverware. It's bright and colorful and easy to hold—who could want more. I want her to keep the skill of feeding herself as long as possible. Again, the saying that you use it or lose it comes into play here. I was always picking something up to try, some things worked and others didn't. Your loved ones needs may vary, but you want them to be as independent as possible for as long as possible.

Your hospital supply store will be a place visited regularly. I learned when I went to get my mom's wheelchair—that there is something else out there. What we got was a "transfer chair". It is primarily for someone to push (which was the case for us). It has 4 small wheels and easily folds up. It is very lightweight. This was just perfect. So there are alternates to the traditional wheelchair. I always have them put a Velcro seat belt type thing on mom's wheelchairs. Learn what's out there and make things fit your needs!

I have also found that having friends over when I'm doing things for my mom has helped me. Friends watching me do things have given me great ideas. My mom's friend's daughter (who worked in a nursing home) was helping me one morning. She said why don't you attach one side of the flaps on the diaper before you pull them up. What a great idea that was! Now I only struggle with fastening one side instead of two when she stands up. Wouldn't you think that I would have thought of that myself? So simple yet it never occurred to me. My cousin told me to switch the wheel section on the front of the walker, so with the wheels on the inside, there is more room to go through doorways. It was a great idea and so simple. Another time one of my friends said, why aren't you putting the support socks on her in bed before you get her up. Again, this was another good idea that I never thought of myself. Keep an open mind—you need to be listening to others; they may come up with good ideas, too. Just because I've done something a thousand times, doesn't mean I know best or the best way to do a particular task. I have been so surprised when these people have told me such useful things. Good ideas can come from the most unlikely place—keep that open mind. Always listen to any suggestion from anyone.

The talents you will develop will be so surprising. I have become very versed on many unusual topics. My cousin called one day asking what I knew about incontinence products. To my total amazement, I found myself talking about the pros and cons of each of the various products that are on the shelves. I didn't even realize that I had been talking non-stop over 20 minutes without taking a breath, until my cousin pointed that fact out to me. Her next comment was that she guessed she called the right person. When did this happen? When did I become an expert on adult diapers? On a closing note, there are many products and one for almost every need. I just want to mention that you shouldn't be too quick to dispose of anything. My mother's bedroom was bulging at the seams, because these packages are big and bulky. I would buy when there was a sale; storage can be a problem. I used to store the extra packages of diapers under the hospital bed, until I got the Hoyer Lift, and then I couldn't do it any longer. Do try to keep them all on hand because their needs will change and the products you use will change continually.

Another talent I had developed was to be able to carry on a conversion with virtually no response from the other person. As my mom's disease progressed, she talked less and less. To my surprise I found myself talking more and more. I didn't want her conversation skills to disappear, so I wanted her to be constantly exposed to talking. These talents you develop may be very surprising to you.

Set up a daily routine

Make sure that exercise is an important part of their daily routine. I believe that diet and exercise go hand in hand to achieving a healthy mind and body. When she was healthy my mother always loved to go for long walks. So we try to walk a little bit every night. It seems to relax her and in some ways I'm sure that it feels familiar to her. We don't walk for long periods of time now—as she gets worse our walks get shorter. But I still believe that the walk is an important part of her day—every day. I make sure that I walk her into daycare daily, so they see me do it and won't hesitate to get her up also. I also make sure that we walk out of day-care daily. I feel that I never ask anyone to do something that I don't do—whether it is at work or with my mom. I certainly can't ask the workers at daycare to walk my mom to the potty, if they think I don't have her walk. At home I don't push her in the wheelchair at all, we walk from room to room. I realize that in daycare, they are busy and can't do what I do, so a comprise has to be reached. I accept that they will do their best—but it won't be like if she were home with me. Financially I have to work and she has to go to daycare and we have to make the best of the whole situation.

A well balanced diet is very important. I watch my mom's sodium and fat intake. I make sure that her diet is very high in fiber to help keep her regular. Prior to my taking care of her, she was very often constipated. We try to eat many fruits and vegetables every day. Luckily my mom's appetite has always been good. If the person you are taking care of isn't eating well there are many liquid supplemental drinks, which provide the needed vitamins and minerals. Remember you can always doctor them up in a blender with additional fat-free ice cream or anything that your person would like. Time for Creative Foods 101—try different things. The good news is that they may not remember what they like or dislike eating now. My mom hated oatmeal. She will eat it for me now and even tells me that it's good (I'm happy, because it is so nutritionally good for her). Creative thinking with their food consumption can and should go hand in hand.

Our nightly routine is very special to me. As with getting up, are getting ready to go down is just as regimented. My favorite time is when mom and I play our version of "twenty questions". If she remembered she would realize that the questions are the same night after night—but she doesn't remember. I want to help her hold on to her memories for as long as possible. I start out with her name. Usually she says her maiden name, but sometimes it is her married name. Then I ask her where she lives. She also tends to remember the street name. My mom truly has an advantage to that, which most people couldn't say. Her whole entire life she lived on the same street. One of the stories that she would tell was that my dad said to her "stick with me kid and we will go places" and she would always say "I did, from one side of Broad Street to the other!" She and my dad moved across the street into her grandfather's house. Her grandfather built this house in the 1860's and this is where my mom and I still live today. So the street name was probably easier for her. I'll never forget that one day, she was having a bad day answering the questions. When I asked her where she lived, she replied, "why right here!" I never doubt for a minute, that she didn't know she was home. On good days, sometimes she would answer me with a tone like, what a stupid question that is. My next questions would have to do with school and usually names of relatives. I hoped by us playing our game that she was able to hold on to those precious memories for just a little longer.

When it is time for a nursing home?

I used to think that there was a specific time that I would realize that I could no longer take care of my mother. Possibly when she doesn't know who I am anymore, or maybe when she doesn't know who she is, or maybe when she can't completely follow directions anymore. I have discovered one important fact. It isn't a question of when my mom is ready for a nursing home. The true question is when I am ready for the nursing home situation. It is strictly and should only be a caregiver's decision. My mom's condition will be worsening every day. I don't believe that some day I will just realize that I can no longer do it anymore. I believe that it is "my" state of mind that will determine when something has to change. It's a horrible disease and the future won't be good. Every day I see a small part of my mom leaving. It's like you have your loved one, but at the same time, you don't. I'd give anything in the world to have my mother back, the way she used to be. The only good thing is that I believe she doesn't realize what is happening to her. Her entire adult life she had high blood pressure, now her blood pressure is normal. All her worries and cares are gone. And I have inherited all those worries and cares and more! There are bad days and there are good days. Her good days are my good days and her bad days are mine also. I struggle through the bad ones and thank God for the good ones. I'd like to say try to find humor in the amusing things she does at times. But in fact, there truly is nothing funny about this disease. I love her with all my heart, and it does break my heart to see how she is. There are so many times, that I wish I could tell her something and know that she really understands what I'm saying. I do always talk a lot; I want her verbal skills to continue as long as possible. My constant babble can and does go on for hours. I have no idea what she truly comprehends, but my chatter is continuous. I am always asking questions and waiting for answers, some times she surprises me. If I ask her what her age is, she will answer with a number. When I ask her what color something is, she will answer with a color, it just isn't necessarily the right number or the right color. I believe the key is to just keep them talking for as long as possible.

It's funny that the things that possibly bother you the most now, you will be praying that they do it later on. My mother had a horrible thing about asking to go to the bathroom every 5 minutes. She wouldn't remember that she just had gone. It used to infuriate me. I would pray that she would stop asking about the bathroom. That old saying of be careful what you wish for, because it could happen, is so true. Now she doesn't know when she has to go. She will sit on the toilet for a very long time and not even realize that she is supposed to be going to the bathroom in the toilet.

Other times I couldn't keep her down; she was constantly trying to stand up. She didn't realize that she couldn't walk without the walker and she would stand up and try to walk without it. Then her leg would give out and she would fall. I would be trying to cut the grass in the backyard and I would see her start to stand. So I would be yelling, "sit down", turning off the lawnmower and running to get up to the porch before she would fall. The only chair that she couldn't get out of was those Adirondack chairs, she would struggle to get out of it and it could give you some time. Both the daycare and myself at home had gotten those chairs for mom. Those few moments of time meant a lot. Who would ever have thought that there would come a day that I couldn't get her to stand up at all? It happens.

My lesson learned is to appreciate what you have at the moment. Live for the present, because today truly is a "present" to you. Don't get down on yourself if you lose your patience, because being a caregiver is extremely stressful. I believe that you get more patience as time goes on—I know I have and I had absolutely none before all this. All the frustration and the aggravation you are going to feel are normal. I found myself just taking a deep breath and trying to regroup. Focus on the moment. Most importantly don't beat yourself up; the word "guilty" should not be in a caregiver's vocabulary.

Take care of the caregiver

Our job is enormous. I know that I am doing two full time jobs and then some. Unless you are in this circumstance you cannot begin to see the vastness of this great responsibility. My world is my mother's world. I know I have said that her good days are my good days and her bad days are mine also, but it is just so true. I love my mother with all my heart, but I have learned the importance of taking care of myself so that I can better take care of her. My mom always got her pills, and I got mine if I remembered and I had the time. My mom always was clean and looked her best; while I did as much as I could in the time I had left for myself to get ready. My mom still comes first with me, but I am actively making an effort to find time for me, too.

At first, I put a chart up on the refrigerator to mark my accomplishments. Each column was all the things I needed to do for myself daily; by marking "x"—s, I could see how well I was doing or not doing. They say if you do it for a few weeks, it becomes habit. I didn't find that to be the case. I did well for a while and then slipped back into my old bad habits. So I find my chart to be vital to my goals. I am trying to watch my diet, drink more water, take vitamins, and get more exercise.

To get more exercise, I joined the Curves that is near my house. The circuit looked easy enough and I felt it was something I could handle. However, the biggest surprise was not the exercise that I got there, but the friendships I formed. It seems that the same people tend to go at the same time and you really do get to know these folks. This physical outlet became also a spiritual one. I never dreamt that would happen. I made many new friends. They even saw my mom on some days when I took her there with me. Mom loved to watch action and us girls jumping around was sure something to watch. Going to Curves helped me stay on track. My feeling better will help me be able to care for my mom much better. This is such an important thing to remember. You HAVE to make time to do the things you need to stay healthy yourself. You need to focus on you.

Recently I was awarded from Erie County, a citation signed by the County Executive, for the second annual "Caregiver of the Year Award". It was presented on November 20, 2003 because November has been named National Family Caregivers month by President Bush. A huge part of me feels very guilty receiving this award. I am doing what my heart says I should be doing—no more, no less. Without the help of the Tonawanda Fire Department, who answer my phone calls with such a gracious attitude, whether my call is once a week, once a month or twice a day. When my mom slips to the floor, there is no way I am capable of picking her up myself (prior to the Hoyer Lift). My mom also has a very sensitive vasal-vagal condition and she would pass out (medical term is syncope) easily. When she would pass out, I would call to make sure it wasn't anything else. They always came here with a smile and a pleasant word. They would always take the time to even talk to my mom. They didn't just offer assistance, they showed unbelievable compassion, and they became our friends. They will have my heart-felt thanks forever. Also, our family doctor wrote a prescription for a medicine that hadn't been approved by the FDA yet. I had heard of a drug (Memantine) in Europe that they had been using 20 years. I did research and showed the doctor. He had written the script, a letter for customs and filled out many others papers—to make it happen. I fought to get that medicine for my mom. Luckily a lady who was bringing her husband to my mom's daycare had instructed me exactly how to go about getting it. It was extremely costly, but we did it. We got that Memantine (known as Namenda) before it was approved here in the states. The first time we got the pills, I was so surprised that the directions that came with the pills were in German. Silly me, of course they would only be in German. Luckily, my cousin could translate so we knew the proper dosage. So I faxed it off to him and he quickly wrote back with the translation. I found you will go to any length and any cost to help your loved one.

I may have been the one receiving the award—but it has to be shared with the City of Tonawanda Firemen and our family doctor. It has truly been a combined effort of all—without them I could never do what I have been able to do for my mom. What a wonderful gift they have given me—those firemen, our doctor, and my friends have allowed me to have my mom at home with me here. There are no thanks great enough for this gift. I may have gotten an award but it belongs to all of us—truly I'm the blessed one.

When I accepted the award I was able to say a few words. I said that nothing I have ever done has been so hard; I have been discouraged, frustrated and some-times totally overwhelmed—but also, has nothing ever been more rewarding in my whole entire life. I believe that our legislators need to look at the concerns of a family caregiver in their home situation. We have needs and they are so costly—wooden ramps outside doors, wheelchair vans that can be purchased used but still are very costly. My used van costs more than I earn at my full time job in an entire year. There is no help from the government. If I had any doubts about what I was doing, they were gone when my mom would look up at me and smile. Was anyone listening? I can only hope so. I have made a promise of myself to accept any invitation to talk to anyone who can help improve the situation of the caregiver. We are the advocates that have to make changes happen. The caregivers are a voice that needs to be heard. I can only hope that someone will hear me and listen.

I had hoped that my citation could somehow make things a little better at work. I had to take time off to go to Downtown Buffalo to receive the award, so work was fully aware of what was going on. Hardly anyone asked me about it afterwards. I took the citation to work and showed it to some of them. Not even two months later, I am still being harassed as to why I'm minutes late getting to work. My immediate supervisor told me that she's seeing others who have children and sick husbands getting to work on time. If I need more time at home, then maybe my job shouldn't be full time, etc. I can't begin to explain my mornings to her. I have to be totally ready myself before I even wake up my mom. In the winter, this means also shoveling of the ramp, just to get the wheelchair out of the house. Not to mention doing the entire driveway if need be. After waking my mom—the daily struggles begin. First I need her to sit up in bed (and stay sitting—not so easily done). She wants to lay back down and go back to sleep. Next, I have chairs on each side of her and I need her to push up on the arms of the chairs. This is usually a make it or break it kind of a situation. At this point we could end up on the floor and I would be calling the firemen. If we end up standing, I remove the diapers and set her on the potty. Then we start doing the sponge bath thing—which she isn't crazy about and she especially doesn't like raising her arms for me to wash under them. So after this struggle, we stand and I continue washing her up. We dressed as we were sitting on the potty. After we are standing, we walk into the kitchen to take our pills and eat a cereal bar. The taking of the pills is the next struggle. Lately, she doesn't want to drink, so I have many choices of drinks available and hope I can get something down her. Then putting on the winter coat is my next struggle. She doesn't like to be bundled up in that heavy coat, but here in Buffalo you need a heavy coat in our very cold weather. Of course, after all this, I can start my 60-minute drive to work. Who knows what the roads hold in store for me. I have to drop mom off at daycare and continue on to work. Truthfully there are many days that I'm amazed I even get to work at all, let alone being on time. But I keep trying and do my best. I really believe that you can only do your best. How work can't be a little more understanding, I will never comprehend. Comparing my mom to a couple of small children or a sick husband is so totally unfair to me. What could I possibly say to a woman who says this to me? All this whole situation proves to me is that they will never understand, and only ones who are in a comparable situation can begin to understand—as I have already said many times.

Life lessons

I have learned this understanding, a first hand lesson from my loved one. My mother has been and is my friend, and has been always teaching me everything I know. She is my best friend and my biggest supporter. She was and still is, a great person and if I can only hope to be half the person that my mom is, I'll be doing fine. She's taught me so much, and the truly amazing fact is she still is teaching me daily even now, so many different things. My most recent lessons include, compassion, patience, understanding and unconditional love. Patience was one of my hardest lessons to learn. I'm the kind of person who is always hurrying and running around. But I now know that rushing my mom is probably the worst thing to do—repetition, talking slowly, using my hands to motion, can help tremendously. You don't learn these things quickly; I believe time plays a huge role in this. A lot of it is a "learn as you go" proposition. The unconditional love was an even bigger surprise to me; she truly guided me to put everything into proper perspective. How was it possible to learn so much from a mom who has lost so much of herself?

I do know I'm changing constantly, I'm not the person I was a year, a month, or even a week ago. I was a person who resisted change all the time and now I feel like I have embraced change and readily adapt to it. Everyday I feel like I'm one of those runners on the track that jumps hurtles as he is running around. My day is one hurtle after another—most times, thank goodness, I'm able to jump over them, occasionally I have trouble and knock one over. This means getting up, setting it up again—and most importantly, to continue running and jumping the next one. These hurtles are sitting her up, then getting her up, then going potty, then washing up, then dressing, then standing, then walking, then taking pills, etc. and on goes my day. Please don't get me wrong, each day is truly a blessing and I thank God for everyday that mom and I have together.

You have to live each day at a time; but when you plan you have to think about 6 months to a year ahead. When I did remodeling at the house, my mom was using a cane—since then we have gone to a walker and then a wheelchair. So when you are making changes or doing any improvements on your house, think of what lies ahead. You may not be using that wheelchair yet, but make sure all doorways are wide enough. I had made a huge mistake with my car. I had a Chevy Cavalier that mom couldn't get in and out of. So I thought by getting a normal full size car (with those child proof locks) that we would be okay and we were—for a few months. Then I had to purchase a 5-year-old used wheelchair van from a place that doesn't take a trade-in. So then I had two vehicles, which really wasn't good, and I had to embark on a new skill—selling a car on my own. What fun! This is something that I had never done before in my life. Had I been thinking ahead I could have avoided the whole problem. Moral of this is to be sure to think long term and anticipate the future when you are doing that long range planning.

Being the sole caregiver is a huge responsibility. It is the hardest thing I have ever done. As I said before, although it is so difficult at times, it also is the most rewarding thing I have ever done in my entire life. There are no words to describe what contentment you can receive in knowing that you have done this. A caregiver is going to find that there isn't much help out there; no one but you will have the answers you will be seeking. It's up to you to do the looking, and up to you to do the deciding. Use any inputting you can get from any source. Follow your heart. Only you will know what to do. The road of a caregiver is a long and hard one, with many twists and turns. Just when you think that you can handle the situation, something new will happen. My mom always said that God never gives us more than we can handle—it sure makes you wonder. There were many times that I truly felt tested. I know how very much I have grown throughout this whole process. I feel like I'm so different in so many ways. This whole thing has changed me and hopefully made me much better and much stronger. I never had children of my own—now I have a 150-pound infant. She is totally dependent upon me. She knows what she wants to do and does it, no matter what I may say or do. I can honestly say that I love her more now than ever—she truly has taught me exactly what unconditional love is. These lessons are priceless. I have been so blessed to have such a wonderful mother, teacher and an example to live by. She was and still is the best. She is my role model. I look at her life and truly wonder how she was able to do all that she did.

My mom had a hard childhood. Her mom died when she was eight years old and she had to help take care of her little brother. She learned to cook and clean very early on. She grew up quickly. She graduated from high school. She wanted to go on to college, but at that time, it was the boys that were sent on to further education—not the girls. She worked full time. She got married, took care of a husband and baby while she also cared for a father that suffered with Parkinson's disease and had dementia for over 10 years.

Probably marrying my dad was one of the best things in my mom's life. He was also a very caring person just like her. My mom often told the story that when my dad proposed to her, she said no. He asked her if she didn't love him. She answered that it was because she loved him that she wouldn't marry him. She told him that she wanted to care for her father, and she wouldn't expect my dad to live that kind of life. He said that it was because he loved her so that he wanted to be there to help her care for her dad. To me this is the most beautiful love story I have ever heard. I was blessed to have these two caring people for parents. My dad passed away two days before Christmas in1981 and my mom was still the strong person she was, but I know a huge part of her died that day. My dad had a heart condition, but it was an aneurysm that took his life. To lose a parent is so hard.

Thinking back on the family stories that my mom always told us, one of them haunts me. Her father (my grandfather) had an older brother named Otto. They said he was a very strange man and one day, he left home and never returned. Whenever an unidentified body matching his description was found, my mom's father and my uncle would go to see. He was never found. Knowing what I know now, I would think that this man maybe suffered from Alzheimer's disease all those years ago. It just wasn't known and didn't have a name way back then.

My mom is a very remarkable person. Some say that our house was always spotless; it isn't now—cleaning is important but far from my top priority. I try to spend quality hours with my mom—everything else can wait. Our time together is the most important thing. Thanks to that used wheelchair van, we can and do everything. She is in the grocery stores (with carts that have those Velcro straps which attach to the wheelchair), the drug stores, the malls and everywhere else we feel like going. We stay busy, we were always busy and that won't change now. I feel that keeping things as normal as possible is so important.

Church was always a big part of my mom's life. If I had any doubts, I truly believe that there is something much bigger than all of us. I would take mom to church every Sunday and she seemed to really know where she was. She would have a relaxed manner about her; you could actually see the ease in her face. She had forgotten names and things, but I couldn't believe my ears when she recited the Lord's Prayer. What a bond she still had with God! How could she possibly remember that prayer, when she had forgotten so much else? As the disease progressed, she didn't remember the words anymore; but as I said them in her ear, she would nod her head, as I prayed. God was still such a big part of her life. She really did find comfort in His house and with His words. You could see the contentment in her face. Everyone in our church was so wonderful. They would all stop and speak to her. At the beginning, mom would nod and speak and smile. These people paid her more attention than others who knew her forever. I will be forever grateful to those special members of our church. They never said a word to us—when she would speak to me loudly during the service or maybe start snoring during the sermon. The people of our church were so nice to both of us. We had our own special spot in back where a wheelchair could sit next to a small pew seat. Every Sunday we were there, back in the corner. I think that it is so important to do the same things as always.

I've been thinking—what must it be like to have dementia? I'm thinking that maybe it would be like being in a foreign country where no one speaks English. Everyone would be talking and you just couldn't understand anything. It has to be very frustrating for your loved one not to be able to communicate with you. Maybe we should always be thinking that we need to put ourselves in their shoes—because some day in the future that may be exactly where we will be. This is a very scary thought. Hopefully they will come up with something to cure this horrible disease. Every year my mom and I walk (well I walk and I push her) in the Alzheimer's Memory Walk. The last five years of my mom's life we participated in the memory walks each and every year. It was something that we could do to help the cause. Remember doing something small is better than doing nothing at all. If everyone does something small, there can be a huge difference in the long run. Do all that you can.

I was so moved watching President Reagan's funeral on the television, that it motivated me to write letters to all my federal and state elected officials—even including President Bush. After watching the funeral, I went right to my computer and sat down and poured out my feelings. A few hours and a few tears later I had my letter. I hope my little letter can maybe make a difference. However, at the same time I was mailing my letter to the president, on a news clip I watched his father, the former president, jumping out of a plane—sky diving to celebrate his 80th birthday. I hope President Bush could relate to my letter, but at the same time I wonder with his father being perfectly "normal" if he could truly understand. I do believe that we need to try to do something to make a difference at all costs. It will make you feel better and you will be helping others. I truly believe that this is a key to happiness. I feel much more content with my life.

I don't think that you really see your loved one getting worse day by day. This past Mother's Day the daycare that my mom goes to gave me a picture of my mom in a cute little frame. It was a very good picture of my mom; however it had been taken shortly after she had began going there. It made me feel badly because it was then that I realized how very much the "looks" of my mom had changed in a relatively short period of time. Also I had pictures of my mom on my computer and it showed mom walking with a walker by herself—that too has long ago stopped. You definitely don't think of these things until something else triggers your memory and you see how things have changed. It is such a fine balance of knowing where you stand, that she will be getting worse in spite of your excellent care, and still trying to make the most of every encouraging sign that God gives you.

The old serenity prayer comes to mind, accept what you can't change and change what you can. I try so hard to have a positive attitude, and it is getting increasingly harder as this horrible disease progresses. I find myself praying more, wanting to go to church more, and just wanting to believe in miracles. I want a miracle for my mom. You need to be realistic and hopeful at the same time. Hope is really all that you have. I want her to be better and that just isn't an option; in truth, just staying the same for as long as possible—is the best to possibly hope for. To stay positive in such a depressing situation is truly a very hard task. The hardest thing I've ever done. Research has to continue and we need to find a cure. This is such a horrible disease for both the person and their caregiver. I do feel that after many years of trial and error, I'm coping better with this dismal situation my mom and I have been placed in. I am hoping that my story of our trials and tribulations is somehow helping you to cope also.

A Look into the Future

I went to a CPA in 2001 to have my income tax done and doesn't the IRS audit me. The accountant had made my mom a dependent on my form. I had never been audited in my life and I always paid my taxes. It really made me feel horrible like I was trying to get away with something. The IRS informed me that you couldn't have someone be your dependent if they are bringing the same dollars into the household. When you look at my salary minus taxes and at her Social Security and small pension together—the amounts are nearly the same. With mine being only slightly higher in the total amount. If my portion had been double hers, then she could have been my dependent. It made no difference that I have to do so much for my mom and our money is pooled together just to cover all our costly expenses. If my mom was my dependent, I could count the cost of her incontinence products; but since she isn't my dependent, she can't count them on herself. This whole thing is so unfair. Income tax laws have to be reformed. My mom is not my dependent, but she is totally dependent upon me. I wear many hats: I am her therapist as we walk, her dietician as she eats, her aide as she is cleaned up and dressed, and her constant companion—yet she is NOT my dependent. Does this make any sense?

On a last note, even though I feel that I've coped, searched for better ways to do daily tasks, tried to keep positive in a very negative situation—there is still the ever-present frustration. It is my enemy and at the same time it has been my driving force. It is with frustration that I relay this last small story: I had my mom at the store yesterday. People looked at me with sad eyes and they say things like "does she live with you?" I want to scream back that yes she lives with me—she's my mom, my best friend and I want her with me always. I can't take those sad eyes anymore. I don't want pity from anyone; I want help in finding a cure. I throw myself into "missions" at work that can do good and help others. I spear head fundraisers and projects that benefit different things, but what I really want is **someone to help my mom**. If I catch the words "Alzheimer's disease" on the news, I'm glued to the television set, hanging on to every word. I want answers and there are none. Frustration has become my constant companion.

Currently today there are over 5 million Americans that are living with Alzheimer's disease. Alzheimer's disease is the most common cause of dementia in older people. One in 10 people over 65 and nearly one half of those over 85 suffer from this horrible disease. Alzheimer's disease is the 7th leading cause of death at this time. Currently there are nearly 10 million caregivers. The experts predict that numbers of people suffering will triple by 2050. These facts shouldn't and can't be ignored any longer.

I want them to find a cure for this disease. I'm one of the baby boomer generation and when we start getting this—it will really be scary. If you are reading this you are probably a caregiver and definitely have your hands full and then some. You probably don't really even have the time to read this. But we need to take time to encourage legislation that can make changes for the future caregivers. The high costs involved with caregiving at home for the individual and the lack of tax laws that consider the caregiver are real issues that need real attention. I think that the key may be to focus on in-home care. It's seems to help both the caregiver and the loved one to stay contented. The cost for the government to keep them at home would seem to be far less than in a facility. Learn about what issues are currently being decided upon and talk to your elected representatives. Please do whatever you can to help make a difference.

Your outlook is the key

I truly believe that how you feel about yourself is the key to dealing with the situation. You have to be content (not, necessarily happy) because this situation is far from a happy one. You know in your heart that you have done all that you can for as long as you can. My cousin is going through a similar situation to mine, she has asked me how I feel. My feelings are—no one loves them more than us. We need to remember that our "worst" days at home may be far better than their best days in a facility. If you are content with yourself and how you are caring for your loved one—nothing else matters. Or should matter, but others can be cruel—words can cut to the core. If only I could live by my advice to my cousin. Many things in life are truly easier said than done. I wish that what people think really didn't matter so much. Especially when they are thinking badly of me—how can it not hurt and hurt greatly. I go to church and pray to forgive others who sin against us; yet when it comes down to the knitty gritty of the matter—I can't. How can I love my neighbor when they think I'm not taking good care of my mother and they are watching my every move? My aunt told me to let go of the bad feelings, but how can you when they are constantly believing and saying things against me. I guess until I can forgive, I need to ignore them. You will run into people that won't understand—that much I'm sure of.

I believe that a different kind of daycare situation is needed. So many people are totally unaware that adult daycare even exists. That fact always amazes me. It is such an important thing and so many are unaware that such a thing is out there. I will share what I have learned. There are actually two kinds of adult daycares. The first step would be the "social" daycare—there will be many more of this kind. The hours will be more of a whole day situation, allowing people to get some respite time from their loved ones—or in my case, allowing me to go to work. This is fine when your person has mild or moderate dementia. When the loved one has severe dementia, the situation becomes very exasperating—they can't participate in all the group activities, but the socialization is still simulating for them. The second kind of adult daycare is the "medical" daycare. The big factor with this kind is that you have to have some kind of medical need (example: like an IV.) The hours on these places are very limited for only 3 or 4 hours a day and the cost is practically double. It doesn't follow that you leave social daycare to go to a medical daycare—usually that wouldn't be the case at all. I feel there is a need for a next step. When someone isn't good for the social daycare, but isn't ready for a nursing home facility—there should be an intermediate daycare. The focus wouldn't be on field trips, but on mastering simple tasks. It would be like going to a nursing facility to spend the day, but still going home at night. They could have more helpful equipment like the hoyer lifts at hand. With all the social daycares out there, a daycare that offers the next step would seem like a good solution. Even in a living type of situation, you would go from a private home, to an assisted living situation, and then a nursing facility. I feel that the three steps are so important to the daycare situation also. I think that someone should come up with an intermediate step.

In spite of everything, it is so important not to lose fact of the most important thing. Each day I still have my mom—is a gift. A very precious gift that only God can give us. I read an email that I used in one of my speeches once. It said something to the fact "that I grew up in the fifties; an age when everything was saved and re-used, long before the term recycle was conceived. With a father who had shoes repaired and a mother who reused aluminum foil, etc. They were always fixing things around the house, e.g., a radio, a screen door, etc.—things we keep! It was a way of life. All that re-fixing, re-heating, renewing, made me just want to be wasteful. Waste meant affluence. Throwing things away meant you knew there'd always be more. Then when my mother died, I was struck with the pain of learning that sometimes there isn't any "more". Sometimes what we care about the most gets all used up and goes away—never to return. So while we have it—it's best we love it—care for it—fix it when it's broken—and heal it when it's sick. This is true for marriage, old cars, and children with bad report cards, dogs with bad hips—and an aging parent. We keep them because they are worth it and because we are worth it." This email hit home for me. It's true that today everything is disposable; we toss things away without a thought. We need to learn to keep things, not discard them. My mom is a "keeper". We need to restructure ours lives to go back into that keeper mode. Let's hold onto those precious things that are near and dear to us and not throw them away so easily.

Music is a big part of our day. Mom has always enjoyed music. It is so important to focus on their likes. I picked up various cassettes of Big Band groups. We would watch Lawrence Welk reruns on TV. To my surprise my mom and I became country music fans. I had often played the old big band tunes for my mom, but I also found her liking the country music on the car radio. It was soothing, and I would see her foot taping along. So that became my favorite music in the car. There is a country music song on the radio now that truly moves me—it's "Somebody's hero" by Jamie O'Neal. It talks of a mother being a hero to her daughter and now life comes full circle and the woman becomes a hero to her elderly mother. My mom was a hero in my life, she did it all and made it look so easy to boot. I can only hope that in some ways I became a hero to my mom. Jamie O'Neal did a concert at the Riviera Theater in North Tonawanda and I was so happy that I was able to go and see her sing that song in person. After the show she did autographs and I was able to tell her just what that song meant to me. It was a very special moment.

Earlier I mentioned those letters that I sent off to several people after watching President Reagan's funeral. I had poured my heart and soul into that letter and I mailed it off expecting to hear nothing in return. One of the letters did make a difference. I have to say that I never expected the Alzheimer's Association or Senator Clinton to fly me to Washington, D.C. because of it. Senator Clinton was having a press conference on Care Giving to inform people of the Ronald Reagan's Alzheimer's Breakthrough Act. Since she is the Senator from New York State, they wanted a caregiver from New York State also. She wanted this caregiver to speak, and I was selected to speak at her press conference.

On Tuesday, October 5, 2004 Senator Clinton was so gracious to me and I will never forget that day or what it meant. I met Senator Clinton in the hallway of the Russell Senate Office Building right before the press conference. It was such an honor to meet her. I saw first hand that Senator Clinton really cared. I also met other Senators who were joining with Senator Clinton to stand behind this Act. Senator Mikulski told me of her own personal struggle with her dad and this illness. They knew and they cared. It was Republicans and Democrats standing together, working together, and supporting this Act together. Their political affiliation didn't matter; they wanted to make a difference. It was so inspirational. It didn't seem real; here I was at Capitol Hill telling our story. It was such a memorable day. My mom went to daycare early that morning, and I got on a plane to go tell these folks about our life. To my mom, that was a normal day. That night when I picked up my mom at daycare, I told her all about my day. I pray that some small part of my mom understood my words, but I'm not sure that she did. It was all for her, and she didn't even know it. I wanted the lives of the future caregivers to be easier than the road we had to follow. Some positive things can come out of a negative situation when you least expect them. Never give up on your dreams or wishes. Write those letters. Don't give up. Follow any feeling you have; it could make a difference when you least expect it.

I would probably be remiss if I failed to mention my latest yearly improvement project. If nothing else, it was to become a truly eye opening experience in many different ways. My thinking was that I needed to be able to get mom into the house as quickly as possible. In the winter, shoveling the ramp and getting her inside took some time and I would have mom sit in the warm van while I hurried to clear the snow covered and slippery ramp. Pushing a wheelchair up a slippery incline isn't easy—trust me on that. The inventor in me saw the problem and looked for a way to make it better. This will probably also illustrate that not all of my ideas were good ones. It was a simple thought, to me the snow was the problem, so no snow no problem. I was going to cover the ramp. A cover, it didn't sound like a big undertaking; boy was I wrong. Projects do help in the fact that you are hopefully accomplishing something good and it gives you something positive to focus on at the same time. Well after calling the contractor and dealing with an architect, things were in motion. Due to city variances I had to appear at a public hearing to apply for sides to this cover. So on Halloween night, my mom, my friends, my good neighbor, my contractor and myself go to the hearing. The only thing I brought with me was a few snap shots of the house/ramp. There were six members that had to vote either for or against my proposal. The bad neighbor was there. She was screaming and name calling, very out of control. She called my house an eye sore—I had pictures. She called my mom a "temporary problem"—I and everyone there couldn't believe our ears. I stayed calm. She showed her true colors. The variance passed unanimously within seconds. There was no discussion at all. I'm sure it was thanks to her being herself, that they felt sympathy for us. I guess there is some justice in the world after all.

So this was to be the final change for the ramp. This ramp was to be totally enclosed. It was a far greater project in cost than I had anticipated. The time frame was supposed to be three weeks and it turned into months. My mom led a life without debt, she was of that generation where you didn't spend money you didn't have. I'm sure she wouldn't have approved of my choices or the fact that we opened a home equity account, which I only used for our "projects". My aunt had said to me once, what is money—it's only money. She always had me look at things differently. She encouraged me with all of the projects. Make things better for both of you now. My aunt, she was such a wise lady and her advice was so precious to me.

I waited about 5 years to get an aide from the County (Senior Services). I was on the list but our need at first was in the morning, and then there were none for that early in the day. As with everything, our needs changed, and later I needed help in the evenings. I was so happy to finally get help. I will never forget when the county caseworker came to the house; she asked me what the aide did while she was here. I told the caseworker that the aide helped me feed my mom, potty her, do the nightly walking and get her into bed. To which this woman replied "but what else?" This amazed me. Those two hours flew by so quickly; it seemed that the aide no sooner got here, and then it was time for her to leave. Many a night she stayed a few minutes longer (on her own) just to help me more because she liked us. I knew in my heart that this caseworker had no real concept of what was going on here. This caseworker had no idea how long it took to do just one little item of our nightly routine. I was so thankful to have finally gotten an aide and unfortunately little did I know that I wasn't to have that help much longer.

Our aide was a trooper and she joined me in my determination to do the nightly regiment, but it was getting more difficult daily. Our aide was great and she became our friend. Every night it was harder and harder to lift mom. I actually hurt my wrist in trying to lift my mom, but I couldn't and wouldn't give up. However, God stepped in and he took it all out of my hands.

I lost my mom on November 28, 2005. It had just been another day. The day started out normal. She had been running a very low-grade fever, but she seemed okay. She had gone to day care and I had worked that day. When I picked her up they had told me that she had a great day at daycare. They said she was better than normal. The aide and I had just gotten her into our kitchen, and I had just started to feed her dinner. I will never forget that last moment. She looked up passed my shoulder (like she was looking at something above my shoulder and her eyes got very wide). It was like she saw something there. In my heart, I think she was just tired out from the long struggle. I know she knew me, maybe not the name, but she knew me. She was always giving me a smile or a kiss, and I don't doubt for a second that she loved me with all her heart. I didn't want to lose her, but I'm glad that she died at her home, in the home that she loved so much. In my heart I know she knew that she was home, even with the severe dementia. I believe that God took her quickly and didn't let her lay and suffer. She did her suffering long enough with the Alzheimer's disease. She suffered little by little, day by day, losing bits and pieces of herself. It was so hard to say goodbye to the mother that meant so much to me. It has been nicknamed the "long goodbye". It truly was a very long goodbye that went on for many years but ended on that day in November right in our kitchen. I was able to have her about 7 years with the disease—but it wasn't long enough. I'm sure that it's never long enough. There isn't a day that goes by that she isn't in my thoughts. Treasure each and every day that you have with your loved one—these are precious moments that can never be replaced.

On my mom's death certificate it reads cardiac arrest, but I wish it had said cardiac arrest due to complications of Alzheimer's disease. It was the Alzheimer's disease that took my mom's life—not anything else. My mom was in pretty good health except for this horrible disease and I really believe that she would be alive now if she hadn't gotten Alzheimer's disease when she did.

Section 3—After

The final chapter

It's not easy to lose your loved one and it doesn't get easier with time. With that being said I continue …

It took me a long time to be able to go back and finish up on this article. My mom and I had such a special bond. I will be forever changed from going through this experience. My mom was the most courageous person I know. Her strong will and determination was unbelievable. Those two things made her so hard to deal with at times, but it was also those same things that kept her going. She had the will to live. She never gave up and she gave Alzheimer's disease the fight of her life. Her "let's go" attitude kept her pushing and kept us struggling along daily. This awful disease may have taken her mind slowly day by day—but it never touched that spirit. She forgot names, places, and how to do things—but it never touched that spirit. She had the will and the drive to fight it and a good fight she gave it. She still is my greatest inspiration because she just never gave up.

I have often wondered, what would have happened if she had gotten any illness other than Alzheimer's disease? Something like Cancer, where you are mentally aware of your surroundings. I am positive that I would never have been in the role of a total caregiver. She would have insisted that I have my own life. What a loss that would have been for me. I needed to be her caregiver. I needed that caring of my mom to make me be me. That person I am now is because of her. My mom never would have wanted to have my life be dedicated to her, but I couldn't have it any other way. In a strange way, I guess Alzheimer's disease created the compromise that we both needed.

I am so thankful for all the support that I had. Without the agencies, the firemen, friends and others standing with me, things would have been so different. Sadly, the Adult Day Care closed only one month after my mom's death. The lease was up and they decided not to relocate. I would have had to take a leave from my job. How blessed was I to have the daycare for as long as I did. They were there when I needed them. What a huge loss this is for the community! They were the best and now they are gone. We need more programs like this, with skilled and caring individuals staffing them, with people who know how to handle the folks with dementia, with a safe environment where clients are nurtured and encouraged, and where the caregiver can leave them without a worry. The McGuire Carecenter will be missed—they have left a hole in our community.

I had mentioned that I lost my dad back in 1981 and that was so difficult. He was a good father and I loved him. He was in awful pain for a few weeks before his death. I will never forget it but I need you to realize how very different it is when Alzheimer's disease is involved. To lose a parent is so hard, but to lose a parent to Alzheimer's disease is totally gut wrenching. I can't emphasize the time factor, to lose them so slowly, bit by bit, hour by hour, day by day, for so many years. To see a strong independent woman become totally dependent upon me for absolutely everything. To lose her, to lose her wonderful stories, and to lose her unconditional love was unbearable.

Stay focused

My personal goal is to keep busy and try to stay focused. I am still taking it one day at a time. It was such a huge loss. I still believe that helping others is the best cure for pent up feelings. I have become active in being an Advocate for the Alzheimer's Association. I have lobbied in Albany and Washington on different occasions. I hope that my caregiving story can impress these aides and or political figures to remember us when issues involving Alzheimer's disease are concerned. My mom is with me on these trips because she is deep in my heart. She is a part of me. She was and still is my true driving force.

I want to mention a gentleman that I happened to sit next to on one of these bus trips to Albany. He was up in age, I'm guessing close to 90. He told me his story and it was so moving. He reached into his suit coat pocket and pulled out a picture. He says to me, "isn't she beautiful?" She was elderly but very well dressed; I even noticed lipstick on her. Then he reached into his pocket again and showed me another picture. This was of a very young woman and he said, this is how she looked when I fell in love with her. They married and had children. She got this horrible illness. He told me that she had Alzheimer's disease for over 21 years. With his eyes filling up, he turns to me and says, "she didn't know who I was" and "she wouldn't let me kiss her—she was my wife and I couldn't kiss her". It truly broke my heart. I will never forget meeting this man or his story. He had just lost his wife, and he was still making the trip to Albany, as he had so many years in the past. I found something that he told me very interesting. Whenever he met one of his elected officials, he would make a request. Come see my wife. Then he told me exactly who did just that over the years. He is making a difference. He is educating those elected officials. He wanted them to put a face with the illness. The ones who went out of their way to meet a woman who suffered with this disease at a nursing home did so upon his request. They saw it first hand thanks to him. This man impressed me and I will never forget him. He is really a person who is getting the message across to others. He has truly educated many in a very remarkable way.

I too wear a picture of my mom especially when I'm going to lobby. It's on the lapel of my blazer. This woman that I know makes jewelry and she created a pin out of some of my mom's things. She told me the type of things she uses, so that I could gather them. I went through my mom's jewelry box for old earrings, her dresser for old buttons, gathered her old watches and other little mementos. I found such contentment in going through mom's things and picking out the special objects. The jeweler used bits and parts of these items and also used a picture of my mom. It is very unique and very special—just like my mom. I never wear it that someone doesn't comment. Which gives me a perfect opportunity to talk about my mother. The reason that I go to lobby is because I want future caregivers not only to have the resources that I had available, but I want them to have more. They deserve it.

Over a year has passed and I am still finding it extremely difficult to find the words. How am I feeling? How am I coping? There is such a huge hole in my heart that will never be filled. It all seems so long ago now—has it really only been a little over a year and at other times it seems like only yesterday. My cousin calls me about my aunt and part of me wants to scream and say "be thankful for EVERY moment—time passes so quickly". She second-guesses herself constantly and I try to remind her that no one knows my aunt as well as she does and no one cares about my aunt more than her. She needs to believe in herself more. It's hard, and it's a tough job, unfortunately I know because I was in her shoes. She needs to cherish every moment.

I miss my mom so very much, and I miss the structured life we had. My greatest discovery is that I took much better care of her than I do of myself. Her life gave my life the greatest purpose. I wanted to be the best caregiver I could and now I feel that my life is so meaningless. I feel so useless. It's now that my own personal struggle is really beginning. I want so to make a difference—to find the reason we were on that journey. Our story may not be the most unique, but it says so much about the changing life that is occurring now. Children and their parents are "trading places". On TV the reality shows take wives and swaps them. Well, there is a true reality occurring in American homes and it is the swapping of children with their parents for the role of the nurturer and protector. People are living longer and it will be occurring more and more in the years to come. Children are the parents now and the parent is becoming the child to them. My loss was so great because I not only lost my mom, but the child she had become to me at the end. She was the child that I never had—it was a special bond.

Create a memory box

I want to share something that a pastor told me right after I lost my mom. He said that we should make a "memory box". The treasures that you put in this box have to have meaning not necessarily monetary value. The items need to contain memories of your loved one. This way it can be tucked away, but easily pulled out to look into it when needed. For an example, I have my mom's toothpaste (kiddy flavor) the empty tube is in there because tooth brushing was a very big hurtle every night. The box also contains the little stuffed dog that my mom would talk to. My loving neighbor wanted to make me the box. She did, and it's wonderful. It's a huge wooden box that she covered with fabric. The outside fabric shows the music lyrics to a hymn I picked at my mom's funeral service. The inside lining is made from one of my mom's favorite nightgowns. She truly made the box with love. My box is overflowing now with various items. On sad days, I can sit with my memory box and be lost in thoughts remembering the other times. It's one of the best gifts I have ever received. Since it is such a great idea, I felt I had to mention it. Making a memory box for someone or just gathering items to put into it—can be such a rewarding thing.

Let me tell you about the changes that I have seen in my workplace in the past year. Luckily the main boss has changed and the current superintendent is a very compassionate man. He showed much caring and understanding. I remember on one occasion that he even did research on adult day cares for me. I wish he had been there the whole time that I was caring for my mom. You need someone to truly care and give you some leeway and support at the same time. I never took advantage of the situation, often taking no or short lunches to make up hours. Had he been my boss at the start, I'm sure it would have been a totally different experience. Now my immediate supervisor, who will currently pass comments to me like "you know how it is to take care of a parent"—still doesn't really know the depth of the situation. Her mother can still live alone in her own apartment. Many days she is late or has to leave suddenly and attend to a need of her mother's. When I think how I was belittled for minutes here or there, how my job was questioned on different occasions, I can't but help to see the unfairness of the whole thing. As I have said many times, until you are in a situation—you never truly understand. The caregiving of an aging parent is stressful alone, but add Alzheimer's to the mix, and it moves to a whole other dimension.

Make people aware

I don't know what it will take for people to realize that Alzheimer's disease has to be addressed and we need to make strides in research for all of mankind. I wouldn't wish Alzheimer's disease on my worst enemy. It is such a roller coaster ride with the moments of hope that you are hanging unto so desperately. President Reagan's death made many people aware of this devastating illness. It took a well-known person that suffered with this illness, to bring it to national attention. We need to move to the next level now. We have made such great accomplishments with Cancer and AIDS, we need to see that someone steps up to the plate and hits it out of the ball park for Alzheimer's disease. Budgets are tight. Everyone is cutting funding and cutting programs. We can't let any progress we may have made come to a stop. We don't want to lose the scientists who are working now, but leave because those research dollars stop. We need the current research to continue. We also need more research and we need that cure. I want a world without Alzheimer's disease. Let's make that vision a reality. Please help in any way you can.

Originally, I just wanted to help others in a similar situation to what I was in. How is it possible that while writing this, my whole mission took a different turn? I want this book to have a dual purpose. First, if you are caring for a parent with Alzheimer's disease, I hope in reading these pages you can understand my life and hopefully find some guidance for yours. Most importantly, please know you are not alone.

There is a much bigger second group that I want to reach. My message is for the people who haven't been touched in their own family by Alzheimer's disease. If you are reading this and luckily are not directly involved in a care-giving situation, I hope you will get the understanding and the compassion to deal with others who are. I want to help to educate you. My goal is to relay stories and ideas and make anyone be able to "feel" this illness. The vastness of Alzheimer's disease is so hard to imagine because it truly is an all-encompassing disease. This not only affects the person, their family, their friends, but even their communities for a huge piece of time. People are living longer and everyone has the chance of getting this eventually, because that percentage increases with the increased age. People are battling Cancer, surviving that, only to succumb to Alzheimer's disease. This disease can happen to us all—the rich, the poor, the healthy, the sick, any color, any race, and not just people over 65—anyone! Alzheimer's disease shows no favoritism and no mercy!

Alzheimer's disease isn't only for the older people. There are a huge group of folks (under 65) who have the early onset type of Alzheimer's disease. It is currently estimated that there are 500,000 people with the early onset form. Their physicians misdiagnose many of these people. This can lead to things like an early forced retirement and possibly making incorrect life choices such as retirement options or insurances. This illness will drastically change their lives, and it will entail an even longer period of time due to their younger age. The cost will be disastrous. Combine these folks with all the baby boomers who will just be getting older and the results will be numbers that are truly astounding in the years to come.

My mom's battle with Alzheimer's disease ended, but I can't let her fight die in me. Once it has touched your life, I guarantee that your life will never be the same.

It is so hard to realize and accept how little control we have in so many ways. I found out that I was **not** in control. The only thing we can control is our own attitude. You need to think positive and continue to hope. Become your own inventor. You are not alone. Dream those dreams and try to make a difference. Above all else, remember to be true to yourself.

Thank you for taking the time to read my story. The writing of this did truly just pour out of my heart and onto the paper. Now I wish to share my journal …

My journal on my mom
—Tracking of Memantine

You need to know exactly where my head was at when I started this journal. I was so frustrated and feeling so helpless. This totally helpless feeling kills you. It is so hard to watch your loved one getting worse day by day. You will do anything—grab for any straw of hope. Someone who brought her husband to my mom's daycare, told me about a drug her husband was on and I asked her how she was able to get this drug. I knew that this woman was driven like me; she would take her husband to a special doctor that was an hour and an half drive away. She tried everything and I wanted to do that also. She helped and guided me and I was focused on getting this drug for my mom. They had been using it in Germany for 20 years. I had absolutely no doubts about doing this. I heard that the FDA was looking at it, but that process can take so long—and time is what we don't have. Time is your enemy. So I did what the lady from daycare told me to do. I did research and took it to our family doctor and he wrote the script. I got the paperwork all together and got it sent off. It would come by International Federal Express. It was very costly, but anything was worth a try. We were fortunate enough to be able to get this drug Memantine before the FDA here approved it in the states. I wanted to track the effect that this drug had on my mom's condition. That thought led to the creation of this journal and with the constant urging of my aunt, it happened. The following pages are the actual journal entries.

Tuesday, June 10, 2003

I want so badly to continue taking care of my mother, but there have been so many declines.

My mom's current condition is not good. The last time I saw our physician; I asked him if she was moderate or severe. He told me that she was in a severe range now. Although I have been able to handle her alone most times, if she slips to the floor from the bed in the mornings I have to call the fire department for assistance. But other than them, I am her sole support.

Her hand to mouth coordination is slipping. I still encourage her to feed herself, but she is having some difficulty. Her standing up is harder and she needs constant verbal direction. Her walking is much worse and continues getting more slumped over as the day goes on. By the end of the day she is almost completely bent over when she walks with the walker. She is much quieter now, sometimes I can't get her to answer me or even look up. We are having trouble going on the potty, constant accidents.

I am hoping for some improvement with this new drug.

Wednesday, June 11, 2003

First day of morning half pill of memantine. She showed no bad side effects of taking the pill. My cousin has translated the brochure that came with the medication (it was in German).

Thursday, June 12, 2003

She seems to be talking more in general.

Friday, June 13, 2003

Mom was holding phone better and was answering questions, which she hadn't been doing lately (said hello and good bye, etc.).

Saturday, June 14, 2003

She is much more alert. Good eye contact when spoken to. My aunt called her from kitchen and she hollered back.

Tuesday, June 24, 2003

Increased new medication—now 1 pill in morning and ½ pill at 2 pm.

Thursday, June 26, 2003

Mom had doctor appointment. She was sleepy. I told doctor that daycare said she is very sleepy for them. He discontinued her Prozac and her respidal. He wants her to go for blood work and he will see her in one month.

Sunday, June 29, 2003

She is still showing signs of being very alert. She looks in direction of sounds—good eye contact. I've noticed that she now responds to Hello or Good-bye or Good night when someone says them to her. She even waved goodbye. She knew her name (as usual), but she also knew my name—which she hasn't known for a long time.

Tuesday, July 01, 2003

She was more awake at daycare today. She is walking much better, much straighter and much quicker than normal. She is very alert again. She talked with sister-in-law on phone. She was holding phone on the ear and talking very well. She doesn't always answer correctly, but seems to answer a number question with a number answer, etc. The changes are remarkable. Today is the first day of two full pills. She is taking the second pill at 4:30 instead of 2pm now.

Wednesday, July 02, 2003

She stood up at daycare by herself today. They commented on how more awake she is there. She talked on phone again tonight—not as clear as yesterday. But she did say she was talking to "Anna" tonight. She has much less trouble standing and is almost walking by herself.

Thursday, July 03, 2003

Mom was tired this afternoon. She was dozing after dinner. She knew her brother's name, her fathers name and her aunt. When I asked her "where do you live"—looking for an address, she answered "in a house".

Sunday, July 06, 2003

She repeated a prayer I was saying at bedtime—line for line.

Monday, July 07, 2003

She knew her brother's name; mother and father's names, favorite aunt and her own name—but she didn't know me. She knew she lived on Broad Street in Tonawanda. Her walking is much better. They said she was tired today at day-care. I put her down a little earlier than normal tonight.

Tuesday, July 08, 2003

I have noticed that mom is answering questions with the right type of answer. If it is an age, she answers with a number, not the right number, but a number. If I ask for a color, she gives me a color, not the right color, but a color. She has waved good-bye on many occasions.

Friday, July 11, 2003

She is walking much better and standing up much better. She isn't talking all the time—but she said a whole sentence today. I was trying to get her to go into her room to sit on the potty. She stopped and said, "I don't want to go in there". I was amazed, my aunt turned on the light and she walked in there.

Saturday, July 12, 2003

She got up and walked into the kitchen. Ate cereal and banana for breakfast and she got sick, threw up and passed out. I called fireman and they said her vitals were good, so I let her rest all afternoon. When I asked her how she felt, again I was floored. She replied, I just don't feel good—my throat hurts. For months she had only done 1-word answers, this was unbelievable.

Monday, July 14, 2003

She is following directions so much better. She had forgotten how to spit tooth-paste water out of her mouth and she is doing it again. She is blowing nose with tissue, I used to say blow and she didn't know what to do. It is so amazing. She is getting up much better and her walking is so improved. She isn't talking as much as she was when she first went on the drug, but she is still talking in sentences when she does. She really seems to have an "understanding" about things around her. She is watching TV, which she hasn't done for months. It's like we have gone back in time.

Tuesday, July 15, 2003

She is doing very well. They said that she didn't eat lunch today—which isn't like her. But she is very awake. Walking is much better—she is actually moving walker by herself. She knows her name, father, mother and brother. Knows the street she lives on. As I was putting her down, I asked her the color of my shirt. She replied, "It's pretty. It has flowers all over it." My shirt does have many small daisies all over it. Whole sentences that are actual observations—I'm amazed.

Monday, July 21, 2003

I'm discouraged at mom's progress. Her speaking is less and less. Her speech was slightly slurred and "nonsense" words with some stuttering. She may have a bit of a cold, so I'm hoping these effects are temporary. This has been going on for three or four days now.

Friday, August 01, 2003

We have out of town company and she is doing great. She seems alert and is taking no naps. We went out for lunch and she did great with her hotdog. She was great at the picnic that evening—smiling a lot. So enjoys being around people.

Tuesday, August 05, 2003

During our talking before bedtime, she is telling me stories. A few sentences together, somebody put something on the floor and she stepped on it so no one would see it—I was amazed. We were talking about school, she told me that she didn't like spelling, but when I asked her to spell Grace she said g-r-a-c-e. Again I was amazed.

Saturday, December 06, 2003

Tonight mom seems very sharp. When I asked her the usual questions I was surprised by some of her answers. I asked what day of the week it was. She answered "Wednesday", when I said it was Saturday; I asked what day tomorrow was. She said "the day after". I put up the Xmas tree today. I had asked mom what she wanted for Xmas and she said, "I want everyone to be happy". What a beautiful thought!

She is definitely talking in whole sentences. This morning she had said that she didn't feel good. After dinner, she had said that she was scared. I noticed that she has said that before, always at the same time of night.

Sunday, December 07, 2003

Last night mom got up by herself and fell out of bed. I couldn't believe my eyes. She was lying on the floor right by the door. Her left arm got the worst of it, many skin tears. This is something she used to always do. She has gone back in time. Closing the door may not be a good idea any more.

Thursday, January 15, 2004

Mom is doing pretty well lately. She isn't as good with her name and address as she was. She is good about first name only and sometimes city. But she is talking more on her own initiative. Example, I put juice in front of her and she asked me, "What's that?" In church the other day she said, in the middle of the sermon, "let's go home". I see complete thoughts and whole sentences much more often than before.

Friday, January 16, 2004

She is much more observant than in a very long time. As we are walking through a room, she is not only holding her head up, but she is looking around the room at windows, open doors, etc. I asked the usual name question, she didn't know her name, but when I asked her to spell grace, she said g-r-a-c-e. She seems to be listening more and responding correctly to my chatter.

Sunday, January 18, 2004

Mom had a very good day today. We went to church this morning as usual. She definitely seems more aware of her surroundings. She ate her lunch by herself and she totally cleaned her plate. She knew her name, street and city today. I asked her at two different times today. The one time she used her married name; the second time she used her maiden name. She told me this afternoon that "let's go downstairs in the basement." When I asked her what for, she said to clean. How could she possibly know how bad the basement is????

Sunday, January 25, 2004

Mom had a sneezing spell at church this morning; she threw up and passed out briefly. She came to and we stayed in church, she was fine afterwards.

She was very anxious that afternoon. Wendy stopped for tea and I couldn't get her to sit still at all. At one point she turned to me and said "Shut up". There a complete thought and very well expressed.

Thursday, January 29, 2004

She definitely seems to understand what I'm saying to her much better. Tonight she called out my name when we got home. When I went through all our usual questions, I then asked what state do you live in and she said "New York". I asked her to scratch my back and she answered, "find your father and ask him to do that". When I had picked her up at daycare today, she was rolling her eyes. I see so much more expression from her.

Tuesday, February 03, 2004

When I picked mom up at daycare, the lady there was telling me that Bill (another client) was singing, "the old gray mare" and there mom was singing "she aint what she used to be". And the two of them were doing this about a dozen times. She said it was so cute—I wish I could have seen it.

Thursday, February 05, 2004

Mom is much more vocal. When we sat on the bed, I asked mom to say the prayer. I asked her what we should thank God for. She said, we should thank God for heaven. I asked what else. She said for our happiness. I asked what else and she said for her mother. My mom never ceases to amaze me.

Friday, February 13, 2004

Mom's second day on the antibiotics for a urinary tract infection. There were 2 bacteria's found in urine sample. No drastic change shown yet. But she did know me, called out my name at suppertime.

Special note—mom is allergic to smz/tmp, she broke out in a rash that covered her body on Sunday, and we never went to church.

Sunday, March 14, 2004

Mom was very alert today. She thanked the deacon passing the wine for communion. He looked surprised that she spoke. I took the wine—and then mom asked the deacon—"what about you?" We both looked surprised at that one. Wendy and I took mom to mall; she ate lunch in the food court and was very alert, taking everything in. During lunch she was talking, smiling and laughing—it was great.

Sunday, March 21, 2004

She had a bad day yesterday. She slept in and wasn't sharp at all. Today she was much better. I left the room to throw a load of wash in and when I got back in the living room, she asked where I had been?

Monday, March 29, 2004

I had a doctor appointment tonight. You can see he is thoroughly amazed at my mom. She was tired, but she still had eye contact and answered. At one point she motioned to the doctor to come here (like you would wave to yourself). He responded and came right over to her.

Wednesday, March 31, 2004

My mom was quite ingenious with her answers to my questions tonight. I asked her, "what's your name, sweetie? She answered—Sweetie. I asked her what she did today. She answered—"what ever you wanted me to do". This is so not my mom—she never does anything she doesn't want to. After our bedtime prayer, I asked her what we should thank God for and she shrugged her shoulders. It's amazing how often she is using gestures to get her point across.

Thursday, April 01, 2004

She is so much more alert. I told her to look at her hair in the mirror at daycare and she did it. She was tired today. She knew her name at bedtime. She spelled out Grace for me. She didn't know her father's name. She told me that she had a brother, but his name was Walter (not right).

Saturday, April 03, 2004

Not a good day. She woke up in a foul mood and it lasted all day. She was struggling getting up out of a chair and she wasn't walking well. She was nasty and swung at me a few times today on different occasions. She seemed very on edge. When we were talking to my aunt, she kept saying, "let's go". When we got home, she was shaking her hands. She ate well, but I'm still having a hard time getting her to drink liquids.

Sunday, April 04, 2004

I've found that her best times are either early morning or right before bed. This morning when I went into the room, I said—I love you mom. She answered, "I love you, too". Her comments are definitely showing some thought processing; she isn't simply repeating phrases.

Thursday, April 08, 2004

When I picked her up at daycare, they told me that she had been very talkative today. So when we got home I asked her if she wanted fish or ravioli for dinner. She answered "no ravioli". When we got done with supper, she told me that "I want to go to bed"; then as if I didn't understand, she said, "I want to lay on top of the bed". When I asked her how to spell Grace, she didn't respond, so I asked what letter does it start with—she answered "K". She told me that her father's name was Al and that was her brother's name. She wasn't good with names, but she was constantly chattering, telling me stories.

Friday, April 09, 2004

Mom passed out this morning. There was no sign it was coming—no throwing up or bowel movement before hand. She seemed to zone out (looking at me, but not seeing me) right before she passed out. It was definitely a little different this time. She had passed out before this same week on Tuesday at daycare also. That time she did throw up prior to the passing out. She answered questions well at bedtime, she knew her name, her father's and mine.

Saturday, April 10, 2004

Mom was so cute at bedtime. When she is on the potty is when we always talk. Tonight she was telling me about someone—"she tells me don't do this and don't do that". I realized that she was complaining about me to me. So I couldn't help myself and I asked her—I bet you don't like that! She answered—"Well no, but what can I do about it". She definitely has the talent to make me laugh.

Tuesday, April 13, 2004

Mom had a doctor appointment tonight. She was so alert. She heard noises around her, which she hasn't done in a very long time. Every time she heard a door sound, she yelled, "come in". At one point she kept saying, "I don't want to sit here, let's go". We are practically carrying on a conversation—it is amazing. When the doctor entered, he said hi to her and she answered "hi sir". It isn't even all the talking she is doing, but also there are eye gestures as she talks.

Saturday, May 01, 2004

My Aunt Anna called my mom to talk. At one point she asked mom "how old are you, Grace?" to which my mom answered "too old to remember". We all had a good laugh on that.

Tuesday, June 22, 2004

Mom hates having her teeth brushed. This doesn't change from day to day. We always do it after dinner at the kitchen table. Tonight, when I said to her "we have to brush our teeth now", she answered to me "we don't HAVE to brush my teeth". And the truly funny part of this statement, she said with her mouth barely open (as someone talks when they have a puppet on their lap).

Friday, June 25, 2004

I am always worried that my mom will be losing more and more of her memory. Last night I was so happy because she answered what her father's name was. And later when we were doing our exercising (walking back and forth) she commented on her "Aunt Gubby". These names are usual, so I know she isn't just saying some name. I do see a decline in her physical motion. She isn't as strong getting up off a chair. When we walk I have to hold the walker from behind with both of my hands.

Saturday, June 26, 2004

My friend Wendy had a big birthday surprise party for me. I couldn't believe how well mom behaved. She always loved people and I still think that shows through. She was smiling and waving at people all day long. When people were starting to leave, she was giving good-bye kisses. It was a little late when we got home and was afraid that I was going to have a hard time with her; but she was following directions so well I couldn't believe it.

Monday, September 13, 2004

In general I have noticed many changes recently. She doesn't always know her first name many days. She knows nothing of her address most nights. She refuses to cooperate getting out of bed in the morning—so now we use a Hoyer lift. I only used it once a day and just to get her out of bed. Tonight she made me very happy, when I told her that I love her, she said, "I love you back". It touched me so.

Saturday, September 25, 2004

I was so happy that she knew her name, first and last today. That hadn't happened in a long time. She is still talking, but often it isn't recognizable words. She isn't taking pills well the entire past week. You fear that these are permanent changes. She isn't eating as well; she tends to put too much in her mouth and is missing the bowl with her spoon. I notice more coughing when she drinks. I need to look into thickener for drinks.

Tuesday, February 08, 2005

She is so alert today. The doctor put her on an antibiotic and she is remarkable. This morning when I woke her, I was talking to her and all of a sudden she said, "What do you want me to do?" She knew she was Grace. When I asked what city she lived in—she said Buffalo. I asked her the color of my eyes—she leaned over and looked right in my eyes and said "blue". I told her, how did I get so lucky to have you for my mom—she smiled at me and said, "thank you". I was able to get her to stand up for me tonight. All in all, it was a very good night.

Thursday, February 10, 2005

After we got home, I grabbed the mail and was reading the Alzheimer's Newsletter and not paying any attention to my mom. She called me "Nancy". I was so surprised. I can't remember the last time that she called me by name. She is always so more alert when she is on an antibiotic—it is amazing.

Friday, February 11, 2005

I'm struggling getting her to stand up. Since Christmas and she hurt her wrist, she won't push up on the chair arms anymore. I am definitely doing more lifting, than she is raising herself with her arms. I continue to do this, because I want her to keep walking—so she doesn't forget how to do it.

Monday, February 14, 2005

She is still on the antibiotic and she is speaking in whole sentences. It is amazing. Tonight she said, "Where am I?" Then she yelled, "Come here". The neighbor next door helped me with mom and when I went back into the room, she asked me "Who was that?" She is so much more alert when she is on antibiotics.

Wednesday, March 23, 2005

She isn't standing up (out of chair) well lately, but in some ways she is doing well. She seems to follow directions better lately. This morning I asked her to sit up straight in the chair and she did. She seems to understand better. I have been giving her a Motrin in the morning and at bedtime. Tonight she was telling me a story and she leaned forward and actually whispered things to my ear. Every night I ask the same questions, and tonight I repeated myself 3 times, she looks discussed with me and says, "I'm thinking". The past two nights I didn't need any help getting her up to walk. Today was shower day and she is very alert on shower days.

Wednesday, May 04, 2005

She isn't standing up at all, no help and it takes two people to lift her into a standing position. She still can walk after she is standing. Tonight she was speaking in whole sentences that made sense. I was giving her soup and she said, "put it down". I was talking to her and she told me to "go ask him (gesturing into the other room)". She still answers question, more often nodding than speaking. She seems to still be aware of her surroundings.

Thursday, June 23, 2005

I took mom for a perm and she was very alert. As soon as we got there, she said, "Can we go now?" She seemed to be aware of her surroundings and asked me the exact same question again (half way through the perm). I was able to stand her when we got home, but I couldn't get her hand off the wheelchair and onto the walker. I have been giving her Motrin at least twice daily for a couple weeks now.

Friday, June 24, 2005

Mom had a good day today also. She told me her name (first and middle). As I was driving home I said that we had to go home and have supper—to which she answered, "I had supper". She always was one to have the last word. It is good to still see her true nature coming out yet.

Sunday, August 21, 2005

Thank goodness that I have help every night getting mom up to walk. But today at 1:30 pm she was trying to stand, so I said I'd help her. She had to move her hand from the chair to the walker and she did. It was unbelievable. We walked from the living room into the dining room and then back to the chair. I had given her 3 Motrin yesterday and some cough medicine today. She seems so much more alert.

Wednesday, August 31, 2005

The doctor has put mom on allegra and nose spray for allergies. She was so sharp today. When I got to daycare, I asked mom what she was doing and she said "waiting for you". There was lots of eye contact and lots of talking. She was eating very slowly and didn't seem interested in the whole process of eating (not like herself at all). The nose spray caused bleeding, but no runny nose tonight at all. At one point tonight, she told me that I looked nice. Very logical thoughts and many gestures with her eyes.

Monday, November 7, 2005

Today was my mom's birthday. She turned 84. We had a small party. The aide, Brenda, Wendy and myself were there. Wendy had made mom her favorite chocolate cake. Mom hadn't fed herself in quite a while. We were all standing around having coffee and weren't paying attention. All of a sudden, we notice that Grace had picked up her fork and was eating her chocolate cake all by herself—we were all surprised.

Wednesday, November 23, 2005

She seems okay but she is running a low-grade fever. I had called the doctor and he said to wait and see if it goes down. It was 99.7 today.

Thursday, November 24, 2005

It was 100.5 today. Today is Thanksgiving, so we can stay home and I can push liquids. She didn't eat well.

Friday, November 25, 2005

It was 98.7 today. Today is a holiday for me, so we can stay home and she can rest.

Saturday, November 26, 2005

It was 99.4 today.

Sunday, November 27, 2005

It was 99.4 today.

Monday, November 28, 2005

It was 98.7 today. She did go to daycare today and I went to work. They told me she had a great day. I had called the doctor from work and she has an appointment for Tuesday.

This was my last entry.

Sorry for all the gaps in days over the years. It was very hard to write in the journal, making time to sit down in front of the computer was difficult.

Wednesday, February 28, 2007

Reading through this now—this journal is very special to me. There are so many small things that you tend to forget. I would highly recommend everyone to take time (as busy as you are) and keep a journal on his or her loved one. I only did this because I wanted to see how the new drug was going to affect my mom. The drug was so very expensive and very hard to obtain at first. I felt that anything was worth a try and did everything I could to make it happen. She took the drug for many months and then we heard that the FDA was considering passing it. Luckily for us, the FDA finally approved it and we were able to get it at the local drugstore with just the cost of the co-pay.

I wish I had written so much more down. You tend to forget the many ups and downs and the details involved get lost in the shuffle. The idea of just writing down moments will be so endearing as you read through them later on. Please learn again from my mistakes and force yourself to make notes now, whether it's on your computer, in a notebook or in a diary of some sort. You won't be sorry that you did. What an addition for your memory box! Those moments need to be saved and savored.

978-0-595-45013-8
0-595-45013-X

www.ingramcontent.com/pod-product-compliance
Lightning Source LLC
Chambersburg PA
CBHW020357290526
45785CB00005B/2330